LIVING
{CANCER}
free

A Warrior's Fall And Rise
Through Food, Addiction + Cancer
— And How You Can Too.

SARA QUIRICONI

↦

DEDICATION

In dedication to my Mom, Dad and Brother, who supported me through it all. Thank you for giving me strength and love, and never letting me give up.

In gratitude to my husband, my twin soul, Javier, who gives me the wind under my wings to keep flying free every day. I love you.

In honor of all of those who will read, and share these stories and learnings with the hope to positively affect lives and inspire a movement to LIVE FREE.

CONTENTS

FOREWORD

I came across the text I'm about to share with you in a Facebook post. This post had over 163,000 shares and 245,000 likes with 37,000 comments at the time of publication. Prior to reading it, I was in the midst of a bad argument with my husband. It was the morning, and both of us were feeling incredibly hurt from the harsh words we had said (truthfully, yelled) to each other in the heat of the moment the previous night.

It was a fight that had built up over months of financial stress. We threw stones and hurtful phrases, threats of separation, moving apart from one another, and even a mention that our relationship was a "mistake." These are words that, while they aren't necessarily true, they also aren't the easiest to forget and move forward from.

Neither of us knew what to say the following morning, except to give each other space to breathe, think and decide truly what each of us wanted—in life, and in our relationship.

Feeling lost, hurt, alone, and still very angry, I didn't know what to do. I've always had that luck where the message I need appears in my life the moment I need it most. The following post I'm about to share was just that—the message I needed in that moment to listen, to learn from and from which I would set myself free.

The article written was titled "A 27-year old died of cancer. Her Final Advice has the Internet in Tears." Embedded within this article was the original post on Facebook from a brave, courageous Australian woman who struggled with cancer, and sadly lost that battle, offering what she knew were some of her last words to share with the world. She knew to make those last words really count.

I was one of many I'm sure that was left in tears as I read this 27-year old's final advice. I'll let you read on below, and decide if you need the tissues as well, but I will first say this: while reading the post, an entire flashback of my life came before me in an instant. The cancer diagnosis, the eating disorder, the people who were there to wipe my tears, the transitional hardships, the moments I learned from, the ones I wanted to leave behind, and the ones I want to create more of in the future—these all flashed in my mind like a flip book saying *Sara! Cut the bullshit, put your ego aside, and go be vulnerable to save what you know matters the most to you.* Immediately, my perspective changed with my husband, realizing the stupid things I said and, deep down, what I really wanted for us.

I wiped my tears, marched down the stairs, tapped him on the shoulder and said, "If I died for whatever reason today, I would want you to know that I didn't mean many of the things I said last night. I love you, and I want to figure out what is going on and keep pushing forward together as a team. I'm sorry."

Lessons like this are—for me—something that happens from life experience.

It's an honor to publish and share with you the words from the late and inspiring, Holly Butcher.* Thank you to her family and close friends for their blessing to publish the following excerpts from her post:

> *"It's a strange thing to realise and accept your mortality at 26 years young. I always imagined myself growing old, wrinkled and grey—most likely caused by the beautiful family I planned on building with the love of my life. I want that so bad it hurts.*
>
> *That's the thing about life; it is fragile, precious and unpredictable and each day is a gift, not a given right.*
>
> *Those times you are whinging about ridiculous things...be grateful for your minor issue and get over it. It's okay to acknowledge that something is annoying, but try not to carry on about it and negatively effect other people's days.*
>
> *You might have got caught in bad traffic today, or had a bad sleep because your beautiful babies kept you awake, or your hairdresser cut your hair too short...your boobs are too small, or you have cellulite on your arse and your belly is wobbling.*
>
> *Let all that shit go. I swear you will not be thinking of those things when it is your turn to go.*
>
> *I hear people complaining about how terrible work is or about how hard it is to exercise—be grateful you are physically able to. Work and exercise may seem like such trivial things...until your body doesn't allow you to do either of them.*

*To read the original social media post in full, visit the resource page at https://saraquiriconi.com/book/resources/

Remember there are more aspects to good health than the physical body. Work just as hard on finding your mental, emotional and spiritual happiness too. That way you might realise just how insignificant and unimportant having this stupidly portrayed perfect social media body really is.

Give, give, give. It is true that you gain more happiness doing things for others than doing them for yourself. It is a weird thing having money to spend at the end. When you're dying, it makes you think how silly it is that we think it is worth spending so much money on new clothes and 'things' in our lives.

Use your money on experiences. Or at least don't miss out on experiences because you spent all your money on material shit.

Try just enjoying and being in moments rather than capturing them through the screen of your phone. Life isn't meant to be lived through a screen nor is it about getting the perfect photo.

Don't feel pressured to do what other people might think is a fulfilling life.

If something is making you miserable, you do have the power to change it—in work or love or whatever it may be. Have the guts to change. You don't know how much time you've got on this earth so don't waste it being miserable. I know that is said all the time but it couldn't be more true."

As Holly said, life each day is a gift, not a given right. Cancer or no cancer diagnosis, we are all mortal and have an unknown expiration date for when our time will come.

The question is, what will you do with your gift of life in the time you are blessed with it?

We can live in fear, regret or (worse) comfort in an attempt to avoid making the most of our gifts. Or, we can realize, actualize and act on our gifts to live free and be our absolute best and truest selves.

May this book be a gift that keeps on giving for each of your remaining days, as an inspiration and resource to live {cancer} free. Thank you for reading and being a part of the movement.

↦

AUTHOR'S PREFACE

"I've been thinking about doing this for a while. To me, writing in a journal is kind of like talking about whatever is on your mind, but instead, you're writing everything. The whole idea of diaries and journals are kind of stupid [to] me...however, now I feel the need to write about my feelings. My one fear of course is someone reading this. My next, is reading this in the future to myself. I know I'll look back and laugh at myself, but for now, all jokes aside."
— January 4, 2001, written by pen in a journal by Sara Quiriconi

My worst fear comes true. Except now it's a dream come true. Thank you, Cancer. Thank YOU for reading.

~

According to the American Cancer Society, Cancer is the second most common cause of death in the US and accounts for nearly 1 of every 4 deaths.

We often think of death as the end of our life, when we cease to breathe, no longer live, and are buried in a coffin beneath the Earth. But, for many of us, death begins so much earlier in our lives. In fact, I would argue that in some cases, cancer isn't the cause of a death, but merely the by-product of the life lived.

I was diagnosed with Stage 2A (possibly 3) Hodgkin's Lymphoma at the ripe age of 19 years old. They were never able to tell me exactly what was the cause of my cancer. What a terrible, tragic event: you're diagnosed with some thing that intrudes into your life, threatens to kill you, and then you don't even have an answer as to why you have this disease in the first place like it's some magic surprise you're supposed to welcome with open arms and say, *"Hi, Cancer! I've been waiting for you!"*

Or, do we.

See, the thing with cancer is, it doesn't just pop up at your doorstep, unannounced, without any cause or reason. Even though, to this day, doctors and medical boards still aren't 100% sure what causes Hodgkin's Lymphoma, or my diagnosis. There were, however, reasonable causes leading up to it that I'm sure played a factor in the disease that manifested its way into my body.

Cancer, like any disease, is like a red flag that something you're doing is seriously not working. It is literally *DIS*-ease in the body, or when your body is no longer at ease. Cancer is one of the biggest, *"HELLO YO! This lifestyle of yours, this mindset...yeah, it's no bueno for you!"* wake-up calls, or perhaps gifts life can give you—if you choose to see it that way.

Fortunately, years after my last radiation treatment, I was able to see it that way. It wasn't fast, it wasn't immediate, and it certainly wasn't easy. But, I'm here today, to tell this tale, with a much more positive outlook on life, greater health habits, and a different perspective on time, relationships, and what success is. If you're ready, I'm hoping you can take the faster route from this book, those same learning tools, and also develop a life of greater purpose and health. It all begins with choice, and that's a power that only we take action on for ourselves, by ourselves.

These days, if you follow me on social media at @livefreewarrior, you know I'm a yogi. Many people today will ask, *"how did yoga, meditation, healthy eating, and a positive mindset help you through the process of cancer treatment and healing?"*

The truth? It didn't. Sadly, I was still in the thick of an eating disorder, eating foods based on caloric amounts, exercising for the burn, feeling mentally more lost than I ever have been, on an emotionally numbing roller coaster. I hated my body, and in pure hatred of my body, I would often ask myself, *"How dare my body put me through this hell. How dare cancer impede my teenage years and social existence."*

The nerve. I felt betrayed. My own system had failed me. I wondered when this sick joke of a nightmare would end. I wanted to wake up and go on with my merry life as I once knew it.

But cancer, and my life, had others plans.

One day, a nurse in my care unit suggested I do yoga during treatment. I scoffed at the thought. *"No way! I want to go to the gym, lift my weights, burn the calories, and hit the occasional tanning bed to keep my bronze."*

Never say never.

Fast-forward eight years and I was in my first yoga teacher training getting my certification to teach others how to move, flow and be at ease with their bodies through the practice of yoga and meditation. Fast-forward three more years and I was enrolled in an online health coaching certification course educating myself. I now wanted to help others, learn how to embrace and incorporate the basics of living and eating for a focused and well-balanced lifestyle.

Shit.

We could say, "could have, would have, should have" and kick ourselves in our own butts for decades on end. Or, take a hard lesson, reflect on it, and learn to share it with the world with the hope that others will take that knowledge and transform their own lives during a transitional or difficult time when some self-care could be of benefit.

Thankfully, I didn't sit too long in the former category and kicked my warrior heart into high gear. I decided to share the messages, lessons, experiences and education I've learned through classes, social media, retreats, workshops, conversations, conferences, and here, in this book.

If you have cancer: this book is for you.
If you have a friend going through cancer: this book is for you.
If you don't have cancer, keep it that way: this book is for you.
If you feel stuck, in any area of your life, and are looking for change: this book is for you.

You don't need to have cancer to read this book, or to gain positive, life-changing insight. Although I now live a healthier lifestyle and live free of the various cancers that plagued my life, I wasn't very healthy in my approach to food, my mindset or my lifestyle from the age of 14 years old on.

This book compiles an autobiographical recollection of my past before cancer (moving through the dark), my life after cancer (finding the light), and a workbook for you, or anyone feeling stuck in similar emotion, or "cancers." In any darkness, there can be a light. I hope to inspire many with this book as a tool to spark the light that leads the way for you to be your own live free warrior.

In addition, this book is a dedication to all the things I wish I had done during that difficult time while going through cancer. I will share what I've learned in between, and what I'm doing now on a day-to-day basis to live my fullest, healthiest, and happiest life, cancer-free.

This book is for anyone who is going through cancer, for someone who has a loved one in the process of treatment and wants to understand more, someone who struggles with body image, self acceptance, clearing out negative people, going through a divorce, a job change, home relocation, and really any stressful transitional period.

Basically, it's for anyone looking to rid themselves of different "cancers" that affect us in our lives, preventing us from living the best versions of ourselves. Through the process of learning to live "cancer" free, I've embraced and implemented various methods that have helped me to successfully live a life of freedom. I now share with you the message of how to LIVE FREE.

All opinions are mine, and the information shared is based on my own experiences, mind, and body, so please use your best judgment and medical guidance when making any serious health choices if this applies to you.

HOW TO READ THIS BOOK

I could have written an autobiography, sharing with you the history and tales that have troubled, shaped and formed my past. Equally, I could have written just the workbook, guiding you with exercises, tools, tricks, and thought-provoking questions that can heal, educate, and empower you to make your own choices about how you can change your life.

Instead, I chose to write both—in this one, single book. Why? Because I believe if you want to offer a solution to someone, it's more powerful if you first illustrate and illuminate the problem. Further, if you want to focus on a problem, it can only bring about more drama, a sense of victimization, and (to some degree) a sense of entitlement. Therefore, there needs to be an offered solution.

This book will offer some light, some insight, inspire options, and offer education. As the title suggests, you'll learn about my fall through disorders, addictions and finally my cancer diagnosis. Then, you'll read about my rise, to upward journey to be where I am today in a much healthier, happier place.

As a guide, I aim to share my experiences, how I've failed or succeeded in my responsive actions, and what I discovered along the way. This book, I hope, will help steer you on a greater path—a path that I wish I had known about at the time I was struggling to find my way.

Included in the book are quotes from old journals I kept during my years of struggles with food, alcohol and cancer. These quotes are included to emphasize the message and to offer the emotions and feelings to you, the reader, in their truest, most raw and honest form.

~

The book is divided into three sections:

Section One guides you through my past, the "first testament" if you will, offering what I define to be "cancers" that were created in my younger years. A recollection and retelling of the history, accounts, and experiences of my life at the ripe age of 14 years old, which was I believe to be the tipping point.

Section Two guides you to the point of light, beginning after my last radiation treatment, what happened in between (it isn't all unicorns and rainbows, warriors), and the moment I decided to embrace the present day, or the "new testament," now living a life {cancer} free.

Section Three is a workbook, complete with the tools, exercises, stories, and (potential) solutions that I've learned from past and present experiences. I want to offer these up to you, the reader, as an accessible means to move forward in your own life. The intention is that you can elevate from the place you're feeling most stuck; and that in the moment you see how you can move through anything; how you can avoid the pitfalls of living through a cancerous moment; and, how to move away from these "cancerous" situations before it becomes all consuming and possibly something more serious, like an actual illness.

Are you ready for the adventure? Let's leap together! There's a free life ahead of you, of health, purpose, freedom and meaning.

PART 1

WHAT IS A CANCER?
(B.C. BEFORE CANCER)

WHAT IS A CANCER: INTRODUCTION

Cancer: 3. "Something evil or malignant that spreads destructively."

— Merriam-Webster's Dictionary

Cold. Hospital rooms are always so cold.

It's like the freshest reminder that death is coming for you. A reminder that it's here, just lurking around the corner, like an over-bearing mother, listening with one ear, waiting for you to take that last breath of life.

The fact is, death itself isn't so bad, or evil. We know from the day we are born that the day we will die is inevitable, but what's really important, what defines life, are the days in between.

There's always a tipping point. A time when something shifts, or changes from within, where a person's life goes from being ordinary, to be extraordinary. Sometimes it's seismic, the tectonic plates shifting creating vibrations rippling outward that break your external shell.

Other times, it's one word, a sentence, or a single interaction that will stick with your soul and eat you from the inside unless your 13-year old brain quickly adapts how to process it.

My personal shift from "normal" to seismic was closer to the latter. I had a very average upbringing, living in beautiful homes, parents who love each other, who never divorced, one brother, Caucasian, middle-class, suburban lifestyle. There was not a worry in the world.

Growing up, I ate pretty normal for the 90's. Peanut butter and jelly sandwiches, the requisite servings of vegetables when you had to eat them, maybe a Pop-Tart, Mom's homemade meatballs, and the occasional Happy Meal. It's what we knew, and ate, back in those days in North America. That was defined as balanced and "healthy."

I always loved fruit, and still do to this day. When I was 4 or 5, during the summers we'd go to a nearby farm and pick fresh strawberries and blueberries. We'd spend hours romping through the fields picking up the best finds of plump, sweet, antioxidant-filled little nuggets. Taking the tractor ride back, I would gobble them all up before going to weigh-in and pay, with evidential proof of red and blue stains all over my t-shirt. I was a guilty berry thief.

I was never that dainty, nor the doll, nor did I dream of the perfect wedding. I played a lot, creating stories and imagining entire sets, and cities. I would re-create dreams through dress-up, drawing with chalk in the driveway, playing house outside in the backyard with rocks, sticks and mud, playing softball and kickball, and in the basement creating school rooms, figure skating routines, and board games.

I loved dressing up for Halloween, playing "actress" and taking on another personae. I was never really a fan of the candy, opting to make-believe a candy store with my brother instead, selling off bags

4

and bits with play money we had created.

I was a creativity machine, storytelling any scene I could stir up using the props, play things, and materials that were within my reach.

I experienced the typical teenager concerns and issues: fitting into the popular group, if your "friends" like you, what boy in the older grade maybe likes you, who laughs at your jokes, being the star athlete in your team sports, learning to deal with changing bodies, boobs, periods, height, weight and—at the bottom of the list at that time in your life—keeping your grades satisfactory.

At 13-years old, I wanted it all. I wanted to be beautiful and looked at by the crowds, liked by the all the groups in school (especially the more popular one, which I supposedly was a part of), get the straight A's, be the star athlete and learn how to be perfect in my ever-evolving body. Even though I was one of the youngest in my grade—I started Kindergarten when I was 4—I was always pushing to be older, more "achieved" and ready to be in the adult world. I was already over this school stuff and kiddie shit.

I tried to please everyone, but it was impossible. I felt oftentimes like I was failing in all areas of my life in my attempt to be perfect. I wanted— needed—to be "good" in this world. And, actually, I was achieving pretty much all of this. So, life appeared good. However, the exhaustion of trying to be perfect in all areas of my life left me feeling like I was failing, or never enough.

Life gets tricky when you place all of your self-value in the hands of others, and on the approval of others. You want them to value and validate you. You lose control and life is anything but in your hands now.

"I remember one night during my sophomore year. I wished

that my life wasn't so boring. Believe people when they say 'Be careful what you wish for.' From then on, my life has been anything but normal." — *January 4, 2001*

Enter: cancer.

A seismic shift occurs. A change in the plates happens. And a pattern of thoughts, actions, and emotions that are anything but "normal,"— as I had wished—begins. My body slowly became disconnected from my mind over the course of the following year, delving deep into an eating disorder, and for the 17 years that succeeded that. I started getting into more trouble at school and with my parents, feeling stuck, controlled, lonely, unheard, misunderstood, unchallenged in school, and completely lost in my own body.

I struggled with an eating disorder, including anorexia, bulimia and body dysmorphia for 18 years. This is something I've come to believe I will have some sort of relationship with for my entire life. I will always question where my emotions, thoughts and actions are coming from when it involves food.

Luckily, today, the eating disorder doesn't control me, nor my relationship with food. I can eat a meal without calculating to the penny how many calories are in it (although, if asked, I could tell you). I'm no longer concerned about where the bathroom is and if it is a single stall or if I have to worry about someone walking in on me if I'm throwing up (although, I still have many nightmares about this). I don't plague myself with the out-of-control feeling of not knowing when to stop eating or if I've had enough (my stomach and my brain have magically reconnected, like a lost high school love, with some much needed time, patience, and healing).

However, the struggle with food goes beyond the actual food itself. It's mental, it's emotional, and it's about control. Food is a substance, like alcohol, or drugs, that provide rewards and after-effects. Food can be incredibly healing, which I will prove to you later in this book. It can also be abused.

The diagnostics and criteria for an eating disorder suggest that the cause of the disorders is a combination of environmental, societal and genetic predisposition. The same criteria (I've been told) can be said for the cause of cancer.

Well, I got them both, so I have to argue that maybe there are some overlying factors between them.

More on my diagnosis and story with cancer later, but for now, let's outline the different factors that define what is a "cancer."

Beyond a disease, as we most commonly know it, I'm proposing to define cancer as:

> *"Any factor that causes dis-ease in the body and/or your state of mind over a prolonged period of time."*

You work a stressful job 70+ hours a week, feeling the pressure to bring in more money. The never-ending demands of your boss, working weekends, and to top it all off, you're missing out on all the things your friends or family are wishing you were a part of. You think to yourself, "I only took on this career because my parents wanted only the best for you." This all leads to stress, inner conflict, and a lack of true happiness. *This is a cancer.*

You struggle with food, toying with your weight for years, trying every diet food out there to get your body to the exact weight that you're seeking, running the extra miles to burn off last night's dinner, and, in the end, you're only gaining weight instead and continue to binge late at night eating the foods you really wanted all day but wouldn't allow yourself to eat. To add to that, perhaps you are like I was and decide to starve, throw up, or employ other harmful methods to rid yourself of calories in an exhausting game of control. *This is a cancer.*

You dream of finding the perfect husband, but just can't seem to stick to the perfect boyfriend. Serial dating, sleeping around, or putting yourself in the arms of someone who doesn't make you feel loved, or comfortable, or who doesn't respect you as a person. Destroying your sense of self-worth, esteem, value and respect, you continue to date, only to find yourself in the same predicament time and time again, just with a different name and phone number. *This is a cancer.*

Starting to see the pattern?

Cancer is anything that causes dis-ease, or un-ease, in our mind, body, and spiritual state. It's a bad relationship, an over stressing, under-rewarding job, a poor mindset and an undervalued sense of our self worth, a false sense of control with food or addictions, or a constant string of diets. It can be any falsified strung carrot placed in front of our eyes that we think if we just keep chasing it, will bring us the great gift of happiness we've been looking to achieve all these years.

Why? Because once we feel that happiness, it will quickly disappear and we, as humans, will be seeking for the next big feat, carrot, or prize. Even if you work 100 hours, your boss will still be asking for more and then guilt sets in for never being around for your family. The goal is achieved, and then you feel you have earned to have a treat (just one treat!) and it ends up spiraling down a rabbit hole of failure (more on this later). The relationship circle is a prime example that what we don't learn from one situation, will eventually show up in life in another. If we think the same kind of guy will fix or heal the hole we feel from within, we will never attract the kind of love we deserve. A messed up mindset of one's self-worth and self-respect will always lead us to the wrong people.

Lastly, in the end, that goal we were chasing—the one causing all of the stress and dis-ease within our minds isn't going to bring about a true sense of happiness and achievement—what is required, is a positive mind shift and lifestyle habits that will keep us living long, healthy and free.

While this book is titled **Living {Cancer} Free**, it's important to start at the beginning where life took a turn and I started to make some of my own life changing choices that, in the end, ended up teaching me some very valuable life lessons that I want to share with you.

Let's take it back to 1999, my sophomore year at Bunnell High School in Connecticut. I'm 14 years old, and old enough to think that I had it all figured out, this thing called life.

CHAPTER 1:
CANCER AS A LIFESTYLE

"Everyone wants the fairy tale, but don't forget
there are dragons in those stories."

— *R. Queen, Darkchylde: The Ariel Chylde Saga*

FRESHMAN YEAR HIGH SCHOOL, 1998-1999

I can never really remember the exact moment anorexia struck, but I remember the slippery slide of a personal challenge to eat less and less gone wrong.

I was a freshman in high school, and a stellar athlete playing the position of lead pitcher for the girl's softball team. When I wasn't pitching, I was playing first base or resting for the remaining innings left in a game once the "win" was secured.

In short, I was the "star" in sports, and that started to become a label I attached to.

High school is always a strange and awkward time. For me, I felt like

I fit nowhere and yet everywhere. I didn't belong to any one group of friends or cliques; I honestly could fit in anywhere at some basic level of comfort.

Not too close, but enough to engage in conversation. It led me to be very much like a chameleon, yet I lacked close connections, which is critical at that age. I didn't have a strong support group. To note, I'm still the same to this day, fitting in nowhere, yet everywhere. Some things never change.

I was deemed "pretty" by genetics, with long light brown hair, kissed by natural highlights from the summer sun, blue-green eyes, average to tall height at 5'7", and slender, by common measurements and sizing. There's a double-edged sword, I believe, when you're deemed "pretty" by societal standards. You are subject to become exactly that—a subject, or an object, for others to either gawk at or tear down.

I became both. Some of the guys in school start to "want you" while some of the girls start to hate you, for fear of competition. Whether you're in high school or not, perhaps you are rolling your eyes right now, agreeing that *some things never change.*

Being pretty, I easily slipped in to the "cool kids" category. Being smart, I easily adapted to the Honors class kids and straight-A crowd. Being an athlete, I easily meshed with the kids on the sports teams.

I always said, one of the best parts of high school was the sports, because it allowed me to focus on the performance and minimize the where you fit "in" or "out." In sports, I had the game to focus on, with less variables to tally in, and like any mathematical equation, I had one of two outcomes: either you win, or you lose.

High school drama brought on by hormones, emotions, cliques, gossip, groups, segregation at lunch tables, eyes on what food you're eating, how much you weigh, if your boobs are growing, who you're fucking, *if* you've fucked someone, what school you're applying to for college, what kind of house you live in, how much money your parents make, do you drive a car, where you park in the parking lot...

High school drama. It's pretty much the same for anyone between the ages of 13 and 18.

How one deals with it all is unique to each and every individual. My methods, apparently, were a learning process that needed a little bit of refining over the years. But, that's life, no?

During freshman year in high school I started to feel this segregation and pull to become an adult, act more grown up and the need to feel "cool" and fit in and be liked by the older Juniors and Seniors at school. It was no longer cool to be playful and choreograph dance routines, and roll on the floor laughing about the stupid jokes you and your best friends were making up into the wee hours of the night—nope, you needed to focus on being more mature and popular.

But the little kid in me never really wanted to grow up. She wasn't ready to be a part of the high school gang. She craved to play outside, indulge in laughter, dress up and spend her time storytelling, and living the carefree life of a kid who could eat anything, say anything, and believe she could do anything.

In essence, that little girl wanted to "live free" in a culture, environment and mindset that wanted to define and label her.

I started to feel torn, trapped, judged, not enough, too much, and everything in between. At the same time, my body was changing, morphing, and growing in weird ways. Boobs and hips became prominent one moment, small hairs on my vagina appeared, and then comes a period and the need to navigate the maxi pad or tampon dilemma. It was puberty—and I absolutely revolted and hated it.

Puberty hit me hard. It was a reminder that I was no longer a "kid." I was turning into a grown-up—whatever the fuck that was at the age of 14. Amidst all these confusing physical changes, I somehow thought I was now a grown-up.

I began to rebel against my body, because in many ways, I felt like it was rebelling against me. I couldn't control what was happening to me physically, and I certainly couldn't control what was happening around me with friends, how others perceived me, liked me, hated me, or judged me.

So, I turned to sports. I then befriended, and fell in love with a lesbian (love number 1).

~

Sex, or puberty, was never an open topic in our household. Although I grew up with incredible parents who supported, loved, and guided me in their best intended ways, when it came to some of the tougher topics such as sex, drugs, alcohol, and even food, to this day, saying words like "vagina" "bulimic" or "anorexia" can close a conversation in 0.2 seconds.

These topics are hard, they're scary, they're "dangerous"—but they're also real.

Len was a year older than me. I was the lead pitcher, and Len was the lead catcher. I was still a freshman, but one of the star players on the Junior Varsity team, skipping the freshman team and starting in JV. I had been playing softball for over 5 years at that point, so truthfully, I was really good. I also had incredibly high expectations for myself, to be perfect, to be consistent, and to deliver.

Len had spunk, honesty, heart and bite—qualities missing in a lot of the girls in high school. *Finally,* I remember thinking, *someone who doesn't want to gossip, or date, or drama, but to just be real, honest, talk about deep topics, laugh until into the night, and play a good fuckin' game of softball.*

For that spring softball season, Len was the catcher, and I was the pitcher. We spent a lot of time together, in sports practice, and on days off we started to hang out. At first, we were just friends. With time, the connection that developed between us and brought me comfort. It was a relief to spend time with someone who shared the same interests as me. The moments I felt down, she was an open mind to share a thought with. I didn't feel judged. I could trust her. In the moments I felt high, we could share a joyous laugh that would linger for minutes on end. And, I believe, she felt the same about me.

Finding her was like finding a golden nugget in a pile of stones. I didn't relate to the stones. But this golden nugget, she got me, she spoke my language. We shared a mutual level of deep, intellectual thinking that could be balanced with humor, sarcasm and lightness from one moment to the next. And, moreover, she accepted me, for who I was. I didn't have to wear Abercrombie clothes, or style my hair in a certain way; nor did I have to worry if she was saying something behind my back to others.

I trusted her. I felt safe.

At the same time, I was dating a guy, a sophomore. I've always connected with older people. Perhaps, the wiser, older soul inside me knew at a young age that there were rings of wisdom wrapped deep within me waiting to be peeled away at the right moment to share.

It was the same thing with this guy, I felt it was the "right" thing and cool thing to do to be dating him, the sophomore, to be accepted by the popular people, go to exclusive parties, get invited to their dances, and to feel a part of the in-crowd.

The difference between these two people I was in a relationship with was night and day. The sophomore boyfriend felt forced, yet looked the part, and the other, Len the lesbian, felt more natural, yet was totally "not accepted" by many. Len was openly gay, and something many people, including our parents, were astutely aware of.

I remember a few "talks" we had, with our parents. It was our parents way of warning us of about the obvious, and to indirectly say it's not OK if you two are together as a couple.

We heard our parents words of concern and warning, deflected the comments in school, and kept on winning most, and losing a few, games on the JV Softball season. The season was coming to an end, and so was the school year. Freshman year almost complete, I felt like I had finally found my comfort zone.

Except, it's high school, and there's really never a comfort zone. Just a series of facades, fakes, cliques, egos, and self-esteems that will rise, fall, or filter out. Everyone is changing and seeking approval from someone else. Nobody wants to be the brunt of a joke, a gossip chain, or the outsider in the sea of fish buzzing around the high school halls.

Thank goodness this was all pre-Facebook, snapchat, and text messaging days. Beepers were the coolest form of connection we had at the time (if you're a millennial reading this, feel free to do a quick Google search to research what a beeper is), but I do remember getting an LG cell phone (not smartphone) once I started driving in my junior year. No pictures, just numbers for dialing. I'm a kid at heart, but still born in 1983.

I remember a moment together, Len and I, in the back of a car getting dropped off after a softball game. We were laughing, giggling, about something in the backseat, and the driver (our coach, who knew us both) was watching in the rearview mirror. Our hands came close, and eventually ended up interlaced together. All three of us in that car that day knew there was an emotional connection between Len and I that went beyond friendship. You could feel it. It was about energy— energy that we could not ignore.

Once summer arrived, there was a lot more time to hang out with Len. I had entire days free, and more time to go to parties, events, and my boyfriend's. At this time, alcohol became present in my life. Initially not a lot, but a sip of something at one party, a glass of wine at someone else's backyard party, and a combination of both at an outdoor party spot we used to go to on weekends in an abandoned parking lot or campground.

Sex also became present in my life. There was no direct outside pressure to have sex, but it did become a subject the boy and I started to flirt around with. Especially because he was older and a part of the popular crowd. I, 14 and younger, was a pretty girl, who now had more free time without school or sports, along with the desire to be accepted in every group and to fit in.

Playing two different "lives" in many ways, I started to become torn, or split, once again, between what was socially correct, and what my inner voice and heart really wanted.

During the summer, Len and I developed a relationship together— as girlfriends. We were kissing, holding hands, flirting and having sexual intercourse as woman and woman. Our relationship became very real, in a time where homosexual orientation was not as openly accepted by society, and in an area where heterosexually was expected.

At some point, I stopped dating the guy, and began secretly dating the girl. The summer was fun because I was spending time with someone I adored and felt accepted by, playing in the traveling softball league, and being free of a lot of the fake bullshit that I happened during the school year. It felt so freeing because I didn't have to try, I just was.

At the same time, however, I still had the other life of being friends with the popular crowd. The friends I've had since elementary and middle school, the ones that (externally) looked like I fit in better with. And this is nobody's fault. It was me who struggled internally and who felt uncomfortable with this scenario. It was me who created the pressure to drink, to go to parties, to date the older guy, to seek the approval of the older crowd. It's difficult at the age of 14 to find your internal voice that says, *"No! This crowd, this lifestyle, and this environment—it doesn't really fit me. It's not me. I'm going to walk away and be in the place that makes me feel at ease and authentically me."*

I'd argue that, even at the age of 29, 34, 52, and perhaps even older, it's a struggle to find that voice. But at 14, when one's self-esteem is low, we're easily (and understandably) confused and seeking external approval. We often feel like we fit in nowhere.

You mold yourself and try to fit in, to seek acceptance, rebel against authority and experiment in new ways to mimic the "idols" of your cliques and community.

You buy the Abercrombie clothes, start to drink, become sexually active, swear, make the jokes you think others will laugh at, talk about the gossip that you think others want to hear, just to prove that you know that "you're in-the-know."

It's the biggest game of bullshit and lies that we feed to our little, insecure, naive minds. To think this type of behavior will reward us with feelings of being happy and loved that we're actually seeking. Perhaps, it's the same bullshit game that many of us adults play when we're much older—but more on that later.

SOPHOMORE YEAR HIGH SCHOOL, 1999-2000

Out with the old, and in with the new. As a sophomore, you're just glad that you're no longer the "newbie" freshman who has just arrived. You, dear sophomores, are evolved. You're older, wiser, and more adult.

Volleyball season began, which I loved. Tall, naturally athletic, and yet I had zero ability to jump, I made a fairly great outside hitter with a serious talent to pass from the back row. Like softball, I excelled at this sport and was quickly becoming a star on the team.

At the same time, I was still juggling the dual lives of being cool, fitting in, and being me: the girl who just wanted to play, make jokes, get good grades, be creative and crafty and excel at sports. The sports and good grades came easy for me. The fitting in part, I was beginning to understand, involved drinking, going to parties on the weekend, and catching the eye of the senior in high school who you heard from the grapevine of gossip that he thought you were pretty.

Being the sporty, intellectual, playful girl came easy. The "being me" part was the tricky one. The latter of the personaes began to be a bit more of a "closet" life, figuratively and literally. People in school, and particularly friends, began asking me if I was "dating" Len, and if we were really together. More specifically, was I gay? I denied any part of it, stating we're just friends, and now bug the fuck off.

I must have been a good actress at heart, because living two different lives and making others believe it is quite a task to take on at 14.

Perhaps I sucked at it, and no one really believed it; but, regardless, it was the life I was leading that very quickly spun out of control.

Remember sleepovers? They were super innocent when you were in grade school, or middle school. Long, late nights with your girlfriends staying up watching stupid movies, eating junk food, painting your nails, or (as we used to) make up really ridiculous stories that would have us rolling on the floor laughing until a mom silently knocked on the door and suggested, "I think it's time to go to bed, girls."

High school comes, and sleepovers begin to be excuses for getting out of your house, drinking, smoking weed, or a way to go to a party and get wasted and sleeping over at someone else's house so your parents don't find out.

First, a few beers, then sneaking small amounts from your parents' alcohol stash, refilling what you take with water, and soon enough, you find someone who is old enough with fake ID to get you booze.

One weekend night I had Len sleep over at my house, and had the grand idea to sneak a full bottle of Dubrof Vodka (or some other poor, cheap alternative) to take some shots while setting up our sleeping spot in my parents furnished basement. One shot, two shots, three shots—I can't remember how many more. I was drunk, the drunkest I had been in my teenage life, but I felt this sense of being free. We started kissing, and making out, one on top of one another, and doing what a couple in love does when being intimate.

A fantasy for, perhaps, some to watch. A nightmare, however, for an unsuspecting mother of a teenager who walks in on her daughter in the arms of another girl under the impression that she is heterosexual.

Drunk or not, I remember flashes of that night like a whipping. Things happened so fast, and all was a blur to me. Len was sent home, her parents called immediately. I was scolded, quickly sent to my bed upstairs, and told, "we'll deal with this in the morning."

"Dealing with" was more or less telling me not to drink, that I was no longer allowed (for many reasons) to be friends or hang out with Len from this point forward, I was grounded, and there would be nothing like this to ever happen again. All the love, sense of security, and feelings of acceptance I had felt being around her were now taken away from me and gone.

I question now: What were my feelings? Why wasn't I asked about how I felt about women? Or, why I was drinking? What was I emotionally trying to hide? What I was fearfully afraid about potentially revealing? But, honestly, who could blame my parents? They were scared, had no idea what to do, and their main goal was to protect their daughter— their little girl—from any outside harm happening.

To be honest, I don't respond well when being told what to do. "Shoulds" and "have-to's" are two words and a part of my vocabulary that I audibly block and mentally ignore when heard in conversations. Far too often, advice or opinions are given that aren't welcome or requested, because we all have our own set of beliefs, experiences, and emotions. And again, let's be honest, it's sometimes easier for a person to fix *or* focus on someone else instead of working on their own shit.

My parents? They just cared. They were, I believe, doing their parental duty, which is having some say or form of authority over a 14-year old daughter. They perhaps perceived this as a form of guidance. It is, however, important to have a safe space where one can share, ask, and be heard. I'm not sure I ever found or had that place at that age.

I remember a conversation I had with my Dad a few days after the drinking and "out of the closet" experience. I was in physical therapy, trying to heal a torn rotator cuff from long hours of softball practice and a volleyball injury. It was a good space to talk with my Dad because it involved sports and athletics—a common ground. It was quiet and just the two of us.

He struggled to find the words. I could tell we were about to embark into awkward conversation territory for a Dad to have with his teenage daughter. How would he approach the elephant in the room—the discovery of his daughter drinking in the basement and making out with a girl? It is weird and difficult.

My father was a man I always looked up to as a little girl growing up. And I still do, to this day. I remember when I was incredibly young, taking some shaving cream, putting it on my face and pretending to "shave" because I had seen my Dad do it. I took up athletics, learning to ski, snowboard, play basketball, softball and volleyball. I was interested in cars, childish humor, and being tough, because that's what made Dad proud.

I could fight and argue and disagree with my Mom until I turned bright red in the cheeks. It would hurt, but our relationship was still manageable. Disapproval from Dad? That was a call for action and change.

Back to the physical therapist and awkward conversation, my Dad eventually asked through stammered words and broken thoughts, **"So you're not...you know...you like boys, right?"**

He couldn't bring himself to say the word lesbian.

It was a moment that broke the anger, the pain and the silence. Together, for the first time in days, we laughed out loud from the tension and awkwardness in the room. To feel his love and acceptance again brought me great relief. And so I replied, **"Yes, Dad. I like boys** *and I'm not a lesbian."*

Clearly, I could say the word lesbian, even though he couldn't.

My parents are not homophobic, racist, or classist, by any means. It was 1999, and being openly gay in high school was very rare in a predominantly white, middle-class suburban town.

And, just like that, I dove back into volleyball, to focus my energy, drown out the emotions and lose myself in something that made sense. Something that was the best distraction, mentally and emotionally. Sports was a place where I felt relatively safe. Movement, I would later learn,—spoiler alert—would be my saving grace for dealing with emotions, stress and unease.

Len and I would pass each other in the hallways, yearning to have a conversation, or an embrace to heal some of the pain. We still truly cared about each other, after all. However, it wouldn't happen. It couldn't happen. So, instead, we passed each other, we attempted to ignore, and keep on while I focused on the other life I was building around me. I felt empty, but kept up appearances. It was easy to be distracted in high school.

I pushed my body hard during that season. I can recall getting mononucleosis (mono), which is also nick-named the kissing disease. Ironically, my volleyball coach got mono around the same time. For the record, we never kissed. There are many other ways you can catch this disease, but its avatar can certainly set the foundation for some enticing stories for the high school rumor mill to spread around like the plague.

In addition, if you aren't familiar with mono, in order to heal from the disease, you're recommended to rest for a few weeks until you recover fully, to prevent complications, in particular, an enlarged spleen.

Taking time off? That wasn't happening for me. I pushed. I was tough and (thought) I didn't need time to heal.

"Weakness is bad; so is crying, acting like a priss and acting like a helpless girl. No pain, no gain."
— *January 4, 2001*

I played and fought through the illness. I could overcome my body's need to rest, because I was above that, and, there was no way I was going to take two weeks off from a volleyball season that only lasted the length of three or four months. Time was precious. Rest could wait.

Eventually, I did heal, and mono, like the flu, made its way in, and eventually out, of my body. The rest of the volleyball season finished. Back to high school drama during the winter until the softball season came around in spring. Sports and movement had helped in many ways, to ground me.

As I already mentioned, I was good at sports, in particular volleyball and softball. My sophomore year, when softball season came around, the coaches of the Varsity Team decided I was good enough to be brought up from Junior Varsity that year. It was time to play in the big leagues with the older kids.

At first, I was excited and honored to play Varsity. A double bonus, Len was already on the team, so there was the potential that we could "sneak" in some time to catch up, laugh together, and support one another without there being a parental voice telling us it wasn't allowed.

My Varsity dreams turned into hours spent sitting on a bench. Being on the Varsity team, and no longer actually playing, began to wear on me. Going from being the star, the leader, the in-demand player as a pitcher and first base, getting all of the action, to then playing relief pitcher, or, worse, sitting out for the entire game was truly awful. This diminished any interest in me to play, any remaining self-esteem I had, and any personal value I felt I could contribute to the team and to the game.

Led by coaches, if I could play or not, was out of my control. Playing softball, as the star, was another thing I loved, and then lost—yet again.

I needed something I could latch on to—something only I could control. It had to be something that I could negotiate on my own terms, to make my own rules for, and be the dictator of in my own kingdom. What did I have on a daily basis that no one could tell me what I should, or shouldn't do, that I could create without anyone deciding anything to me?

Food.

CHAPTER 2: CANCER AS A NUTRITIONAL DEFICIENCY

"Hunger and fear are the only realities in dog life: an empty stomach makes a fierce dog."

— *Robert Falcon Scoot*

SOPHOMORE YEAR HIGH SCHOOL, 1999-2000

An eating disorder came into my life just like a snowball forms. The issue of anorexia or an eating disorder begins as snowflake. You have a thought, in your mind, a little curiosity to see what happens when you start to eat a little less. Diets are always trending, so it's fairly normal in society to "cut out a little of the fats" and begin to "watch your calorie count" or maybe "skip a meal in the morning"—just to see what will happen.

This becomes an issue, however, when this tiny little snowflake of a thought eventually builds into an 18-year snowball of a struggle that never really has the capability to melt its way out of one's life.

No one wakes up one day and decides, ***"I'm going to be anorexic*** *and stop eating."* It's gradual, it's emotional, and it has the power to completely strangle any sense of freedom to live your life in mental or physical peace.

Further, no one wakes up one day and decides, *"OK, I'm over this thing of anorexia and I'm going to go back to my healthy lifestyle again."* It doesn't work like that.

> *"I finished the book [Wasted, by Marya Hornbacher]. It put me at ease to know she's 10x more fucked up than me. 15 years of dealing with that stupid shit [of anorexia and bulimia]. That sucks. I know I'll be fine."* (For the record, I was still throwing up 18 years after I first developed an eating disorder—that sucks.) — May 7, 2001

It is possible to wake up one day and change your mind. I'm not discrediting that. That's exactly what happened when I decided to quit drinking. One morning, cold turkey, I decided I didn't want to live that buzzed, confused, numbed out life anymore.

Food, however, doesn't really work the same way, mainly for the reason, you need to eat in order to live. It is very possible, if not healthier, to live without alcohol. You can go a day, a month, a year, without drinking and still function perfectly well.

Food isn't as black and white. In fact, food is the grayest of areas when it comes to deciding what is optimal on an individual level for the healthiest, longest survival on this planet. You can't just cut out food without another system going into disarray. You also can't cut it out without disconnecting the body from the mind to override our natural instincts to survive.

> *"When I was over at my friend Audrey's house about a week ago, I said that I didn't have any boobs. She told me that I*

really had a bad body image. In a way, she was right. When I see myself, I want to be 3 inches taller with a C cup, thinner thighs, smaller hips, thinner arms, and a flat stomach. The mirror doesn't lie, and I am hardly ever pleased with what I see."

That is where the **dis**-connection, the **dis**-order, and the **dis**-ease start to take form.

END OF SOPHOMORE YEAR, BEGINNING OF JUNIOR YEAR HIGH SCHOOL, 2000

"My sophomore year, around the middle of softball season, I thought it would be 'interesting' to lose some weight. I wouldn't eat breakfast, starve through lunch, go to softball practice without eating, and then go home to eat some of dinner. Of course I lost weight, but I didn't think much of it...I didn't lose that much weight, because after a while, you can't take it anymore. You have to eat."

High school gives you choices. There are options. Do you want to be a part of the band or the basketball team? Do you wear jeans and a blue hoodie, or a short skirt with a button-up top on Friday? Do you really want to go to biology class today, or do you weasel your way out by getting a pass to the nurse? Do you choose the pizza and fries for lunch, or do you want to eat nothing?

With the lack of my participation on the softball team, I needed to involve my head with something deeper. Food, and my control over it, suddenly held incredible appeal. This challenge to control what I ate and my weight lured me in like the smell of the bakery section of the grocery store pulls you in to "BUY ME, BUY ME!" Or, in the case of an eating disorder, says, "BELIEVE ME, BELIEVE ME."

There was no exact moment, but one day, lunch went from being whatever I was bringing to school, to buying whatever was the lunch special, to being a plain roll with butter—nothing more.

In retrospect, it's such an odd choice. A buttered roll: refined white carbs smeared with hydrogenated fats. So poor in nutritional value, yet it was my lunch of choice for weeks on end. Something I remember enjoying was the methodical, meditative process of peeling apart the roll, one flake of crust at a time, eating it piece by piece, flaking off tiny bits of the bread with little dabs of butter. It became a ritual, one that became slower and took longer to consume as time went on.

The roll with butter transformed to be just a roll, and soon enough the roll was gone too. Calorie counting was the next level of achievement in this process. A stellar student in mathematics and sciences, I was always good with numbers. Counting calories seemed like a natural fit to keep my mind focused, in control, and absorbed.

I started bringing my own lunch in an effort to keep the calorie count under control. By packaging and planning out my meals that I brought, I could easily count the calories in a neat, organized manner so as to not have any surprises of my intake.

> *"Today:*
> * *1 Dannon Lite 'n Fit yogurt - 120 calories*
> * *1 apple - 90 calories*
> * *12 pretzels - 140 calories*
> * *1 5-pack of sugar-free gum - 15 calories"*

The worst part of what is written above is that even though that list was written 17 years ago, I can still recall all of those the caloric values in my mind like no time has passed. "It's like you have calorie Asperger's," as mentioned in the movie, *To The Bone.* And, it's true. You can look at a plate and whether you want to or not, your mind still calculates the calorie count like a CPA during tax season. That information never leaves your brain, even when you want it to because you no longer need to reference it years later when you are recovered.

Being vigilant about my caloric values was a way to manage to eat less—to reduce what I consumed on a daily basis. It became a personal test, of some sick sort, to see "what if" I didn't eat all of the pretzels, or what if I just had a pack of gum throughout the school day (which I did for a few weeks).

With my mind fully absorbed with the control of my food intake, it became easier to lose control over the fact that I was no longer the star on the softball team, or that I felt completely uncomfortable around the group of friends I was hanging out with, and that I was no longer allowed to be around the one person that made me feel safe, normal, and loved (Len).

With such a drastic calorie deficit, I lost a lot of weight, and very quickly, It became obvious towrds the end of my sophomore year that something was up with my eating and emotional health. What was reassuring for me, at the time, was that summer was around the corner and then I could easily dodge the plethora of rumors circulating in the high school hallways as to *"Why is Sara getting so skinny?"*

> *"During the summer, it got worse. I would go the entire day without eating, or eating very little, and then eat at night. I only went one day without eating anything. By the end of summer, I weighed 106 lbs. That was the lightest, I think [so far], I ever got."*

Summer allowed me the space to continue to slim, cut, chop and slender my plate—and my waistline—to be perfected in the way I wanted it. The mirror became a friend and a foe at the same time, offering me a secondary voice in my head that unpleasantly whispered, *"You could cut back a little more here, no?"*

I attended volleyball camp that summer. On the upside, it gave me some grounding, moving my body again and being active in sports. On the downside, I was surrounded by people I knew from my high school team, and they were acutely aware of my rapid weight-loss.

My period had stopped and I was kind of happy about it. I never really liked it because it reminded me when I did get it how repulsive the female form and figure made me feel at the time.

By the time school started up again, it was very clear that at least 20% of Sara had disappeared. Volleyball season had started again, and we were only a few weeks into the season. It was also clear that I didn't have the same energy as I had once before, and was struggling to keep up with the rest of the team surviving on little-to-no food.

"At one volleyball game at the John Law Volleyball Camp I fainted. Everybody noticed—my doctor, coach, nurse, parents, and friends—they were all worried. Except me."

I was given an ultimatum. Gain weight, or I couldn't play.

Strike two for the sports teams. I quit.

Life was now, I believed, on my own terms. I hated (and still hate) being told what to do. I was in control, and I would make the rules of my own game, even if it meant leaving behind something I really enjoyed.

"Fine," I thought. *"If I couldn't excel at sports anymore, at least I was pretty and could work towards becoming a model."*

Thin. Tall. Slender. Perfection. Beauty. These all became obsessions. Now that sports were out of the picture, I focused solely on my looks. I dreamed of growing to be 5'9", which would qualify me to be tall enough to be a model. Getting thin was easy, but growing taller? Hmm... how does one do that? I was always just under the 5'7" mark, and that dream of growing taller requires an important thing: food.

What a paradox: I was depriving my body of food to get thin, and wishing to grow taller, which required nutrition (in the form of food.) This equation doesn't work for the human body, nor the mind.

~

One morning I was called in to the school nurse's office to have a pep talk about my sudden weight loss—an intervention of sorts. I hated these types of talks. I was weighed, height taken, and basic measurements observed to check my overall health. I did not divulge to her that I was suffering from an eating disorder. I also didn't share with the nurse that I was eating any differently. Who the hell was she to know any of my business anyway? No way I would share any details with her.

Oddly enough, they sent Len to the office to talk with me. She later told me they asked her to try and get some answers from me because they assumed we were friends. Even though we weren't "allowed" to be talking, I remember that feeling of relief, like I could have a space to talk honestly, openly, and truthfully with someone who actually gave a shit.

Len straight up asked me, ***"What the fuck are you doing, Q?"*** It was the exact no bullshit conversation that I missed so much with her.

I sat there in silence. I honestly had no clue.

No longer playing sports, I started working part-time after school at my family's ski and snowboard store. Here and there, I was still sneaking a few sips of alcohol from my parents' stash, or bumming off of someone else's bottle of whatever hard liquor I could swig from at a party. I craved the "numbing" effects and mental silence. I just needed a little break from the eating disorder constantly pissing in my ear, like an annoying, humming mosquito that won't go away.

As my eating disorder worsened, I became very isolated from my former friends and schoolmates. Always an honor student, I continued to get good grades, but it was very evident that perfection had taken a bit of a wrong turn. Having an eating disorder is a full time job, one that you must attend to on a moment to moment basis. It consumes you. Almost all social gatherings involve food. When you cut that portion out of your life, and you start to be the odd one out, isolating yourself from others. Your eating disorder is your new BFF. We—you and your BFF—have a body to control and put in order.

"What is this little bump on your neck?" asked a kid to me during a study hall period. He was massaging my shoulders and felt a little pebble on the left side of my neck about 1.5" above my collarbone. *"Ah, it's nothing. Let's call it a bean,"* I replied.

From that point forward, the bean was born. Even though, at the time, I didn't think much of "the bean," I had a hunch it was something more. Perhaps, even, did this have anything to do with my eating disorder?

What you attempt to control ends up controlling you. By cutting out so much food in my life, developing categories of "good" and "bad" foods, and having a black and white mentality, the food was now controlling me.

The starvation periods during the days more often than not turned into binge sessions at night. Nights were tricky because I was alone, there was silence, and I had to listen to my own mind and body whether I wanted to or not. Or, eat, to numb it all out.

A food binge is a lot like alcohol, in its ability to numb out certain parts of the thinking brain, creating a calm, soothing affect on the mind.

I would sit in front of the little TV we had in the kitchen at 10, 11, or even midnight watching whatever half caught my mind's sleepy interest. Sometimes it was a movie, more often, the television classic Golden Girls. The main focus was on what I was going to eat next.

Pop Tarts, coffee cake, pasta salad, left overs from dinner, pretzels and peanut butter...anything that I wasn't "allowing" myself to eat or were labeled as bad foods. These were off limits. Even though my anorexic mind had been trained to override my body's signals for hunger, it was still a work in progress for my mind to override my thoughts about food.

Damn! I'm so weak, I'm a pig, I'm disgusting, I'm fat, I'm not enough. These were the ugly thoughts running through my mind throughout the day.

The worse part was waking up with the feeling of an incredibly full stomach, churning and trying to digest the massive amount of food consumed the night before. To this day, if I eat too much, or too late at night by default, the slightest taste of that acid in my mouth in the morning is enough to bring all of these memories (nightmares) alive.

This spiral of hatred towards one's self is a recipe for disaster. That delusional sense of pride that anorexia gives you—that, I can do "without" and "I don't need" is painfully overshadowed by the disgust and grotesqueness of binging and overeating.

I started to gain weight. I was almost back up to my weight before the summer I lost it all. In every way, I felt like I was TOO much: too intense, too loud, too awkward, and too big. I wanted to be small again, to shrink, to hide, and to disappear in a physical way. I had already emotionally withdrawn from life; it only made sense to make the physical remove itself from the social picture as well.

I needed a new method—one that would bring me back down to my idealized, smaller size. One that I could use to keep up appearances that I was "just fine" and be able to hide my weight-loss secret from the world.

Bulimia was the answer.

Maybe it was in an article I read, perhaps it was in a movie or a TV show; somewhere along the way, I learned that you could get rid of food by throwing it up. A person could purge, and not keep any of that food in the body—a light bulb moment of sorts.

If this subject is new to you, a binge/purge episode has two phases:

1. The binge, or consuming a large amount of food in a short period of time

2. The purge, or removal of the food via throwing up or laxatives (I never used the latter, only the former.)

Back to mathematics, I looked at the equation as such—calories in then equals calories out. And what goes in can then come out. This new strategy could even the playing field. One addiction traded for another. Anorexia was quickly replaced by it's evil twin sister, bulimia. Bulimia was the answer to all of my inner struggles at the time. I could eat, consume, and indulge in anything I desired. All of this achieved without the guilt, or the shame. No more feeling fat from over-eating after starving myself. It was a win-win situation.

Of course, it doesn't really work that way. The body absorbs calories that are consumed during a binge/purge episode. Metabolism is the process by which your body absorbs calories. Digestion begins in the mouth with chewing and the combination of saliva. On to the stomach, digestion continues where food combines with stomach acid to break down proteins. In the small intestine, fats, carbohydrates and proteins into glucose, fatty acids and amino acids. Glucose and amino acids are absorbed through the small intestine walls into the bloodstream. Fatty acids are absorbed into the lymphatic system from the small intestine and eventually reach the bloodstream near the heart.*

"It's such a gross, disgusting cycle that one gets caught up in. In the moment you think, 'Wow! I get to eat all of this food! And then it's easy enough because I can then get rid of it all!' However, afterwards, you don't feel so good because that part of your brain tells you that what you just did was wrong. But, you're still hungry, you're still hungry the day after, that night, the next morning, and the binge/ purge cycle will continue. Until you try to stop, and then you've lost control and you can't stop.

"The shitty feeling stays with you all day because you don't know how many calories were absorbed and your mouth tastes like vomit, your stomach knows that what happened was fucked up, and you've messed it up once again. You hate the feelings and the thoughts and the loss of control, yet you do it again. Why? Because no one is there to stop you. Nobody knows but you."

---

* I was later diagnosed with Lymphatic Cancer, which may be related, or completely unrelated. Either way, I feel there is some coincidence here.

JUNIOR TO SENIOR YEAR HIGH SCHOOL, 2000-2001

This secret diet of mine continued behind many closed bathroom doors, running showers at night, after meal "excuse me's" and elected solitude. If you chose not to eat, that was weird. But, choosing to throw up your food after a meal? Socially unacceptable and completely just downright disgusting. Even though bulimia can be traced back to before the Middle Ages, it still wasn't acceptable to be tossing your cookies as a weight-loss method in public. (Good thing.)

There were many days and times where I chose to hide, to duck out of the school social crowd, hang low, and exit my own self out of the picture. The deeper I went into hiding with my eating disorder, the more secluded, alone, and isolated I became.

My parents are not stupid, and were well aware of what was going on. My mom shares stories now of her memories placing her ear up against the bathroom door, listening in to "find me out" for throwing up. No doubt it was scary for a mother, and infuriating for a teenager struggling with an eating disorder.

I still wake up from nightmares. Because an eating disorder is a nightmare. I'm in a bathroom trying to throw up. Sometimes I'm lost trying to find a private bathroom. Other times I'm in there and fearful to be found out. The worst times are when I try to throw up and nothing comes out.

Today these are my dreams, or my nightmares. In the past, sadly, this was my reality.

~

I was seen by at least four different psychological therapists for evaluation and help. Diagnosed Bulimia Nervosa with Anorexic tendencies in the DSM-V (Diagnostic and Statistical Manual of Mental Disorders, Fifth Edition), it wasn't that hard to figure out. However, getting me to comply was another story.

I was stubborn. Let me rephrase that: I am stubborn. I don't like to follow anyone else's rules but my own, I trust very few individuals in the world, and I don't want help unless I'm asking for it.

In a way, I was asking for help. Eating disorders are a physical expression of emotional and mental health that needs guidance, love, attention and self-awareness. The reality was, I wasn't yet ready to heal or get help.

So, I lied. It was easy. Comply, and nod my head. Say yes when I needed to. Make up food stories of the complete meals I had diligently consumed. Eventually, I ended up in a therapist's chair—someone who didn't buy all of the bullshit. This therapist gave it to me straight—the real talk that I needed and secretly longed for. She had short, red hair, a Romanian accent, and a sharp, yet kind manner about her.

Therapy kind of worked, and it got my weight back up to a regular level where I was able to go to individual therapy sessions on a weekly, or bi-weekly basis instead of 2-3 times a week for outpatient group therapy.

I hated group therapy, having to listen to everyone else's struggles, issues, problems, and the same bullshit I was living. It was a painful reminder that "You are sick! You need help!" Fuck, I wasn't nearly as messed up or as thin as some of the other girls. Why the hell did I have to be here?

Group dinners were terrible. You sit at a table together, sharing a meal, eating what you have chosen from the selective, fat-filled menu. My first night at a group dinner, they offered me a turkey sandwich...with mayonnaise. To this day, I abhor mayonnaise. Something about the texture, the smell, the flavor—all of it. But, no one believes that you don't like a food that has "fat" in it when you're in an eating disorder clinic. So, I had to eat it.

I took the sandwich apart piece by piece, like I imagine the Apple store takes apart your iMac when you need to add an extra hard drive. I scraped the pieces of bread and surrounding lettuce on the side of the plate removing any last trace of mayonnaise that was within sight. Then, I began to eat. When I looked up, the jaws dropping and wide-eyes of the people at the table said enough.

Like I said, I ~~was~~ am stubborn.

~

At the same time, I started seeing a guy who I ended up falling in love with (love number 2). He was older, and he worked at my family's store, had a keen interest in sports and possessed the playful spirit of a child. I knew I'd fall in love with him, but being with an older guy, I didn't know how that would go over with my parents after Len.

Pat brought light, company, support, pain, and love into my life. He was my first real boyfriend. We shared a lot of laughs, a lot of growing pains, and spent almost five years together. He knew about my issues with food, and while he didn't fully understand it, he supported me in my efforts to recover.

I was now a senior in high school, and somehow managed to get enrolled back on the Volleyball and Softball teams for the Fall and Spring season. I'm fast-forwarding a bit, but there's much of the same happening throughout senior year regarding the "cancers" that were probing my life. Bulimia mixed with drinking, parties, sex, lying to stay out late, and the self-hatred of all of it fueling the destructive flame.

Graduation arrived, and I was a high honors student and graduated 13th in my class. Grades mattered, sports mattered. And regardless if I was still throwing up, I looked perfectly fine from the outside.

More often than I care to admit, looking "fine" and "normal" from the outside are enough for society to think, "she's OK." What nobody knows is what goes on behind closed bathroom doors, or within your own body below the skin.

I was accepted to every college I applied to, and by the time graduation came, I was more than ready to get out of my parents' home, go to school, and grow up.

Let's get the party started.

CHAPTER 3:
CANCER AS A MINDSET

"90 percent of our physical toxicity is emotionally derived."

— David Simon, M.D.

"It's so strange to me that food is so wonderful to everyone else. But, to me, it makes me feel so depressed. When I'm under stress, it always relates back to food somehow. Whether I'm trying not to eat as much, or I'll eat everything."
— February 27, 2001

Self-destruction always starts out fairly innocent. No one starts starving themselves with the intention to develop a way of thinking and lifestyle habits that will affect every meal and bathroom visit they have from this point forward in their lives. One that could lead to cancer, erosion of the teeth, or (even more fatal, which I am fortunate to not have experienced) heart failure or even death.

"I'm just going to skip this meal for a few days, see how it goes, to lose a few pounds until this "chunk" in my stomach goes away."

You don't realize what you've done until you're crying on a bathroom floor, eyes bloodshot from tears, dehydration and throwing up, or you have a heart monitor attached to your chest wondering if it's within normal range or a signal meaning it's cancer. Worse, your thoughts of suicide and wanting to disappear become so real and apparent that when the words accidentally just "slip" out of your mouth, and you see the reaction in people's faces, you quickly catch yourself, and in desperation, say, "Just kidding."

No, I wasn't. There were moments where I didn't want to be alive. But in the beginning, the game of playing with life, just to see what happens, is just that: a game.

What if...?

What will happen if I try...?

Just this one time...I think?

All of that questioning, thinking and feelings of self-hatred and anger about myself had started to take form. The battle with my body had begun.

What begins as a personal challenge or goal can quickly spiral out of control and envelop your life. Anorexia was hard, and there were many moments where I caved, binged and I overate. Any person who has struggled with an eating disorder, has been over-weight, or has had a substance abuse problem can tell you that moment of caving creates unbearable feelings of shame and self-hatred.

"Imagine looking in the mirror and thinking you're disgusting, thinking you need to be thinner, thinking when and what you're going to puke up. Well, that's what I dream about. I dream about being thin and someone else...I don't want to

throw up. I'd rather drink."

And, that's exactly what I did.

FRESHMAN YEAR COLLEGE, BOSTON, MA 2001

Pat and I moved up to Boston together. More specifically, I enrolled as a Freshman at Northeastern University as an undergrad studying marketing, living in the dorms, and he moved to a neighborhood just outside the downtown area. He worked, I went to school.

I was free. FINALLY! I could make any decision I wanted and do exactly as I pleased. I could choose what food I wanted to eat, if I wanted to eat. I could also choose which party I wanted to go to and how much I wanted to drink.

Vodka was my drink of choice, with Fresca, keeping the calorie count low. The roommates I was assigned to stay with ended up not being so friendly or accepting of me, or my decision to be out of the room as much as possible. Three girls in a cubicle room—it isn't designed for freedom, self-expression, personal space or getting along, it's designed like that for the university to maximize their bottom line.

We ended up getting in to arguments, the two of them against one, throwing accusations in my face. I had had enough when they called my parents telling them I was never there and my boyfriend hit me (he never laid a finger on me, no person has). I was pissed, and decided to have nothing to do with either of them.

At that point, I pretty much moved out of the dorm and moved in with Pat. For the sake of getting to the actual cancer diagnosis in a timely manner, I'll keep this section short and informative.

I drank too much. WAY too much. This wasn't the first time I was drinking, by far the worse yet to come in my life; however, not the worst, nor the last episode of being an alcoholic. In this first go-around—college attempt one, as I like to call it—I was drinking almost every day, missing classes and falling incredibly behind in my assignments.

This had never happened to me before. In all of my high school antics and eating disordered struggles, I had never dropped a grade or fell behind in a course. I was overwhelmed, out of control, and on the verge of a breakdown.

I called my parents.

"Mom? I want to come home."

It didn't go over so well at first, but a parent always wants to do what's best for his/her child. Even if it does cost them $10,000 in the process for a dropped semester.

I left college, feeling like a huge failure. While all of my other friends I had graduated with from high school were still away, as planned, at college, I was back at home. I felt like I was being punished. Of course, I went back to my eating disorder and throwing up to handle with my low self-esteem and lack of purpose and desire to take responsibly for my own issues and life.

Throwing up, once again, gave me the option to forget the pain, the feelings, and the emotions. I was lost, incredibly lost. And, not the good kind of lost you can experience when you travel to find out who you really are. This was the kind of lost that leaves someone with a lack of will to live, to pursue any dream, or to wake up in the morning and even live your life.

I worked, once again, part time at my family's store during the winter and enrolled part-time as a student at Fairfield University, which i could commute back and forth to from my parents' home.

Pat, eventually transitioned back to Connecticut, and our brief Boston stint together had come to an end. We still dated, both a bit confused, angered, frustrated, and knowing things needed to change on both of our ends to survive—in our relationship, but mainly in our own lives.

I was consumed with guilt and shame, feeling lost, stupid, and like I made the biggest mistake of my life that had spiraled out of control. Had this all happened because of an eating disorder? How did this spiral of bad fate and poor mistakes lead me up unto this point?

Fast forward, I started seeing my therapist again, the one I was seeing before leaving to go away to Boston. I saw her on and off on an as-needed basis. Insurance didn't cover her services, so at $300 a session, if I wasn't in need, or I wasn't open to hear and receive the therapy, it was money better saved.

Honestly, no amount of therapy can help a person if he/she isn't ready to get better. On the one hand, I wanted to heal. Dropping out of college, failing in a big way, and starting up again where I left off was a big wake-up call that things needed to change in order to make something better of my life.

On the other hand, I had this thing that I was attached to: an eating disorder. And we (the eating disorder and I) had developed a relationship in that time that kept me safe, in control, at ease, and it was my go-to when I wanted to call my anxious mind. If I couldn't drink anymore (cancer as a mindset) I could at least still cling to my eating disorder (cancer as a nutritional deficiency) for life order and control.

One week before my 19th birthday, I picked up a fresh journal and started writing again:

"A year has gone by, and it seems as if not much has changed. The only differences: 1. I'm completing my first semester (3 classes) of school, 2. I'm one year older...I still want to go away to school...even [my therapist] said I would benefit being on my own. One week from today it's my birthday!

"Two weeks from today I need to get a physical. I am not happy about it. I guess I'm afraid if they tell me something is wrong. After my parents believing that I'm doing SO much better [with my eating disorder] (I am, in fact, doing better than before), I'm afraid to fail."

With writing, reflecting, and thinking more than speaking, acting on, and impulsively doing, I began to see my thoughts a bit clearer written on paper. I began to realize that something needed to change now, or something worse than an eating disorder would happen. This dis-ease of a dis-order in my life was causing chaos and confusion.

Looking back now, reading through my notes, I hear a very anxious little girl looking to control the world around her, seeking to map out each step to know what's coming next, to be the most efficient, organized and "perfect" she could possibly be.

However, there are some things you can control and change in life, and others you need to accept and learn from. Was I ready to learn? Was I ready to grow?

Ready or not, here it comes.

CHAPTER 4:
CANCER AS A PHYSICAL DISEASE

"Illnesses hover constantly above us, their seeds blown by the wind, but they do not set in the terrain unless the terrain is ready to receive them."

— Claude Bernard, 19th-century French physiologist

"My, how things change. One minute, you have school, life decisions, snowboarding and an all-consuming eating disorder on your mind. The next minute, (hold your breath), you also have cancer to deal with. This past week has been hell; a hell, which entails blood tests, CAT scans, and biopsies. I've been diagnosed as a victim of Hodgkin's Lymphoma disease." — January 2003

A few lines later in my journal, after this shocking news is revealed, I'm back to writing about throwing up and what I'm going to eat for the day. Apparently, one dis-ease doesn't stop for the introduction of another.

Not when your first cancer (the eating disorder) is the main control of your current chaos (the real cancer). *Dis*-connect fuels the *dis*-order, and together, they fuel the *dis*-ease.

I found out about cancer after a follow-up pediatric doctor exam. As I had intuitively feared, something was terribly wrong. There was a problem—a golf ball size problem. The little "bean" that was in my neck a few years back had expanded and grew over time. I didn't think much of it, but evidently the bean had grown into a golf ball that was a cancerous lymph node growing rapidly in my neck.

Who knew.

Before leaving for my appointment, my Mom pointed out that I had a growing lump in my neck—she wanted it checked out. I went by myself to the exam, as my Mom was caring for her father who was battling lung cancer at the time. Imagine, a woman caring for a Dad and a Daughter with cancer simultaneously—now you know whom I get some of my strength from.

A benefit of being back in Connecticut and not being away at college in a newer city, was that I was still seeing the Pediatrician I had grown up as a child visiting. Thankfully, Pediatrician offices have a much lighter, more colorful vibe than the adult ones.

By the way, why don't we, as adults, get fun wallpaper, bright decor, and coloring books anymore in the doctor's offices we visit? Adult doctor offices are always plain walls, gossip magazines and the depressing news playing on some big screen TV positioned on a wall with the volume so loud it pierces your ears.

Back to the exam—the doctor checked my neck, palpated it a bit, felt around, asked a few questions, and said I had to go to Yale New Haven Hospital immediately for a test.

Her reaction was a bit alarming, to say the least. Doctors never share too much information—for liability reasons—or what could be or couldn't be, and nothing is ever definite. What was definite was that I needed a few tests and exams right away.

One phone call to schedule in an immediate appointment, my Dad left work and picked me up, and two hours later we were in the waiting room of the Radiology and Biomedical Imaging section of Yale New Haven Hospital. Ironically and fortunately, it was the same hospital that I was born in so they already had me in their system; a real time saver—yay.

I was scheduled for a CAT Scan and a biopsy in the area that was enlarged on my neck. When we called my Mom to let her know where we were and what was going on, she immediately fell to the floor and started sobbing in disbelief.

We all have different emotional reactions to shock. Our emotions differ based on different circumstances and mental triggers. Some cry, some get angry, some get depressed—and someone with an addictive personality, like myself? I numbed.

I went on autopilot mode in that moment, numbing out any emotion or feelings of shock with a big *"...?"* in my head. I couldn't wrap my mind around what was going on, and probably I was shutting out the reality that I actually could have cancer. *"This is just a bump, it will be nothing. They'll drain it out, and I'll go back to my normal life of figuring out what school I'll be attending later in the year, my relationship with my boyfriend, and getting rid of this eating disorder thing. I'll be fine."*

The mind is powerful, and can overcome many things, even the physical needs of the body, as I proved while being anorexic. However, in these circumstances, the body can't always overcome—not that fast.

After the tests, my Dad and I returned back home, waiting (impatiently) a few days for the results. We received a phone call from the Pediatric Oncologist (whom I was referred to by my pediatric doctor) who said to come back in to the hospital to review the results. Doctors don't typically give results over the phone, as this can increase a person's anxiety with potentially life-threatening news hanging on the line.

My Dad, Mom and brother (my entire family) went in together to hear the results. We were placed in a large, glass walled, secluded space to wait until the oncologist could see us. It may have been minutes, but it certainly felt like days. All to sit and wait to hear your fate.

Finally, when she came in with clipboard and a manila folder full of papers, she delivered the results. I'd be lying if I said I remember anything aside from the words "You have cancer." That's about all my ears took in and my mind was able to process in that moment. From then on, everything else was a ringing in my ears that drowned out any other voice in the room. I remember the faces of my family, eyes wide, jaws dropped, tears, and looks of disbelief. I remember how freezing cold the room was. I remember the smell of rubbing alcohol, something that I developed an intense repulsion for. And, of course, I remember my weight that I was admitted in at:

> *"Can you step up to the scale, Sara? 127 pounds," the nurse shared out loud.*

> *(In my head) "Do I really weigh that much? What a pig."*

With cancer, I was pissed, angry and still in some form of shock and denial. Further, I was heavily involved with an eating disorder that still consumed majority of the thoughts in my mind.

My journal read:

> *"It's in Stage 2A, which is good (in a manner of speaking). The lumps in my neck and throat were actually not from the [eating disorder], which is what I previously believed, and therefore, I never made mention of it [at the hospital]. Well, fuck me! This sucks. I felt no fear; just fucking pissed off! Tomorrow I will meet with the doctors at 1pm to decide my treatment. I don't (won't) loose my hair!"*

I did lose my hair—almost all of it. So much of it, in fact, that I barely had enough left to even qualify as hair towards the end of my treatment.

The medical records note:

"Past Medical History:

1. Inguinal hernia repair, age 5.

2. Eating disorder. Upon questioning of eating disorder, the patient became teary and refused to discuss it. The patient does note a history of anorexia and bulimia treated as outpatient. She denies laxative use. However did indicate that she is continuing to induce vomiting, but refused to discuss this diagnosis further."

I remember what I was thinking—I felt violated in so many other ways. They've already tested, poked, and given me my life sentence for the next year or for who knows how long. Now they're going to further investigate my issues with food? Fuck you. I wanted to be left alone, given privacy, and everyone just back the hell away from me.

Coping mechanism: push away. Deny. Shut down.

Upon meeting with the radiologist for initial new patient consultation, the charts read:

"The patient refused to disrobe for physical examination."

The patient. Not "Sara" or Ms. Quiriconi. The patient. And, hell yeah, I refused to disrobe. I'm not a guinea pig. I was 19-years old and feeling void of physical and mental boundaries in every way.

Still in shock and denial, I didn't write another journal entry until three months later.

~

In the interim:

• My official diagnosis was eventually Stage 3A Hodgkin's Lymphoma as noted in my charts on August 13, 2003. In the beginning, they weren't able to decipher whether a spot that had showed up on a CAT Scan on my spleen was scar tissue from Mono or if it was from the cancer. Charts show Stage 3A as diagnosis.

• I was authorized 2 rounds, 4 cycles each, or 8 treatments total of ABVD chemotherapy, followed by a series of radiation in my neck, chest, and abdomen area.

• I had a bone marrow test done so they could ultimately determine the extent to which the cancer had spread. I opted out of Novocain, which typically leaves me feeling depressed, and used only local anesthesia. My reason? I wanted to go to my Spanish class at the University later in the day. I gripped my Dad's hand like a champ while the oncologist jumped, leaped and wiggled the giant needle into my right pelvis while I lay face down. To this day, a bone marrow test is the greatest pain I've ever felt, yet I never wanted to admit that pain to anyone.

• I had a PICC (Peripherally Inserted Central Catheter) placed in my right inner, upper arm (where there's now a "sankalpa" sanskrit tattoo symbolizing determination, strength and purpose). A PICC is a thin, soft, long catheter tube that is inserted into a large vein that carries blood into the heart, typically used for long-term intravenous (IV) antibiotics, medications, blood draws and chemotherapies.

- I still had my boyfriend, who was there (for the most part) to support me through my treatment. Things weren't perfect, but I can only imagine what it's like dating someone in your early 20's who has cancer. It's a lot to go through at such a young age.

- I cut my hair to chin length early on, in the case it fell out, so I wouldn't have to see my mid-chest length locks fall away to nothing. The less noticable the better.

"Some researchers think that infection with the Epstein-Barr virus {also known as Mononucleosis] sometimes causes DNA to change in B lymphocytes. In some cases, this can lead to the development of Reed-Sternberg cells, which are the cancer cells of HL [or Hodgkin's Lymphoma]."

Hm.

However, *"Despite the advances in knowing how cancer cells work, scientists do not yet know what sets off these processes. An abnormal reaction to infection with EBV or to other infections may be the trigger in some cases. But a lot more research is needed to understand what causes Hodgkin lymphoma."* — American Cancer Society*

And, that was written current day, 2018, and I was diagnosed 15 years before that. They didn't know the exact cause then, and they don't know the exact cause now.

*https://www.cancer.org/cancer/hodgkin-lymphoma/causes-risks-prevention/what-causes.html

I was urged to slow down, eat well, rest when needed, and put all my energy towards healing.

I signed up for part-time classes, continued going to the gym, went snowboarding and surfing when possible, hit up the occasional tanning bed (ugh, I know), and continued to count my calories and binge/purge almost on a daily basis.

Cancer didn't scare me; it was just *in the way* of me living my "normal" life.

APRIL 2003, STRATFORD, CT

> *"Cancer sucks, but I'm loving life. Hopefully, by July my life will be normal again. 4 chemo treatments down, 4 to go. Next is radiation. My [white blood cell] counts were too low again this morning, so I'm going back Thursday to get chemo. Every day I pray and thank God I still have my hair. I've gotten to the point where I'm sick of all of this shit, and I'm ready for it to be over."*

During one of my first visits in to the Pediatric Oncology section for chemotherapy, I remember one of the attending nurses or staff ask me, *"What kind of cancer do you have, dear?"*

I replied, *"Hodgkin's."*

"Oh, that's a great cancer to have!" was the reply.

Asshole. What cancer patient honestly believes their cancer is "great" while they're going through a diagnosis and treatments?

Before I was administered my first chemo, the nurses and oncologist shared with me exactly the name of the treatment I would be receiving along with a heavy list of the potential short, then long-term, side affects. Think of any TV commercial for prescription drugs and multiply that list by twenty.

The conversation went as follows: *"We will be administering 4 complete cycles of ABVD. 200mg in total of Adriamycian to start for today, which is this red-colored liquid right here in this bag. Some of the short-term effects are nausea, lack of energy, loss of hair..."* and then my mind went blank. I didn't want to hear it. My ears rung, my mind went numb, and I blocked every single word out after that. I remember them asking me something along the lines of, *"Sara, are you hearing us? Does that make sense?"* I just nodded my head. I didn't want to hear any of it. It was too real.

Loosing my hair was probably one of the most traumatic parts of the cancer treatment.

I was terrified of losing my hair, and I'm guessing I'm not alone in this one for those going through treatment. There's an identity that goes along with who you are, what's accepted, what's "pretty" or normal. There's also a clear, red sign that someone is very ill and sick when their eyes are sunken in, their skin pale, and there is barely a sprinkle of hair on their head at the young age of 19.

> *"I hate washing my hair. It's really depressing, watching it fall out. I thank God everyday I still have what I do [left]."*

In addition to the PICC line:

> *"Too bad I won't wear a t-shirt or sleeveless shirt because of this thing on my arm."*

Along with giving myself daily injections:

"Yesterday I had to learn to give myself shot injections of Neupogen[®] to increase my white blood cell count. As much self-harm that I have inflicted on myself in the past, I still do not like the idea of sticking my leg with a needle."

And, of course, there was my eating disorder:

"I didn't eat sweets or too much all day. Then, at night, I had to ruin it. My teeth hurt all day [from throwing up the night before], so I didn't eat much. At night, I ended up eating more than I planned, which led to poor eating yesterday, and then eating too much crap last night. Today, it's raining.. It looks outside how I feel inside. I ask God, how he can make something so pretty on the outside have such an ugly inside?"

Chemotherapy treatment numbers 5 and 6 rolled on. My hair continued to fall out, so I continued to cut it shorter—by myself.

My Mom and I visited a wig store earlier on in my treatment. I tried on a few for style, size, and mainly feel. I hated it, we started crying the minute the first one touched my head, and we quickly left. I never wore a wig. As embarrassed as I was for being "sick" I also saw it like a body of armor and a battle shield of strength—warrior courage. Maybe I could handle being bald.

All the hair! It drove me crazy feeling them on my skin. The way the hairs would get stuck in parts of my tee shirt as they fell from head and tickled my skin, or get caught in between my breasts in my bra. It was itchy and uncomfortable. To see all of the fallen soldiers on my pillow in the morning or on the headrest of my car after pulling the e-brake and getting out was completely and utterly painful. It was a constant physical reminder of my illness, death and disease.

My Chinese pediatrician urged me to look into drinking this special blend of authentic pure, green tea to aide in my treatment and recovery efforts. A strong supporter and believer in both western and eastern medicines, she thought it would be beneficial in killing off the cancer cells in addition to the western treatment of chemotherapy and radiation.

When I mentioned this to my Pediatric Oncologist, that I was drinking green tea in an effort to help fight against the cancer, she scoffed, *"Well, I don't recommend it. But, I don't think it would hurt."*

Hm.

Her exact words in my records read:

"I believe that Sara is adding green tea to her chemotherapy regimen, and I have no objection to that as long as she follows through with her other treatments."

"I believe," meaning I don't want to fully admit that I heard or approve that.

Now, I do believe I am here, alive to this day, typing these words to share with you because of the chemotherapy and radiation treatments. I am thankful for our modern advances in treatments and studies to cure and kill cancer cells. However, I think it would be beneficial for studies in the United States and for western doctors to be more open-minded to natural methods that could aide and assist, making a western treatment less toxic for long-term side effects, and make the current treatment more potent to kill only the cancer cells.

My oncologist wasn't intentionally stern. However, my feelings for her were a combination of my feelings of hatred towards cancer, and her lack of empathy or emotion towards me. For an oncologist, I imagine you see multiple cancer patients going through similar regimes, check-ups, scans, and treatments each and every day. I am a name with a number on a chart, and I am placed in your care to be best dealt with to reach the ultimate goal of being free from the disease that is cancer. You maybe look at me like a Pac-Man game, using the chemotherapy as Pac-Man and my cancer cells like the food it needs to devour.

Except, I'm not a number, and this is my actual LIFE, and, hopefully not, my impeding death. I am a human, with emotions, and fears, and doubts because this is my first time dealing with any of this. It's left up to me, after the battle of killing off my cancer, to deal with all of the potential negative side effects of treatment in the remaining years of my life. Protocol seemed to override any form of emotional intelligence for my oncologist.

Notice, I haven't mentioned yoga once here in this book so far. Many times, in interviews, it's assumed that I started practicing yoga while I was going through cancer, as part of my healing regime. Nope. A nurse suggested I try yoga during one of my treatments. My answer?

"No way! That's too boring, slow, and not a workout!"

At least she tried.

I started to practice yoga after I was laid off from my first job out of college (spoiler alert) and I needed something for exercise that was local, affordable, and that could burn some calories.

Had I taken up yoga at this point, perhaps it would have helped in many ways, both to aide in the course of chemotherapy, but mainly to heal the long-broken connection between my mind and my body, with food and with alcohol.

In any case, movement always helped me to feel better, and elevated my mood, Whether it was sports, the gym, or being outside.

"I always feel so good after the gym. Refreshed, and today, I feel worked!"

However, with chemotherapy, cancer, an eating disorder, and self-loathing, there was still much more pain than good:

"I have a lot of pain inside of me. I just cried for the past half hour, in between [episodes] of throwing up. Screaming through tears, the pain, thoughts, feelings, and questions that make me unhappy. I shouldn't be unhappy, but there are a lot of things I need to change.

"Yesterday was a blur. Chemo days are always a blur because of the drugs they put me on for anxiety. It's like being drunk without the slurred speech or the alcohol, and minus the laughs with your friends. There is no fun to it. After, you sleep, and later wake up having no recollection of your memory.

"Throwing up is so gross, and the dry feeling left on your tongue is your constant reminder all day of what you did."

Initially, I was coursed for eight chemotherapy treatments. However, just like in life, doctors offer no guarantees. And, neither do chemotherapy treatment outlines.

"[My oncologist] told me I might have another 2 courses after the next one. That would mean I wouldn't be done until August! If I already feel like I'm alone and have no support because everyone else is too busy with their own lives, how will I make it until August? I want my life back!"

Wake up, Sara. This IS your life.

At this point in the chemotherapy game, I started to lose steam. My energy dropped, so did my hair, and so did my weight.

> *"I saw [Lauren] at the gym today, and one of the first things she had to say to me was, "You're so skinny! You're tiny!" Even after telling her, 'Yeah, I know, I know. I need to gain some weight' [Liar. I didn't want to gain weight]. She doesn't know I have cancer."*

Sick or not sick with cancer, losing weight was always a reason to gloat when someone noticed. It was that coy feeling that I couldn't express on the outside but was jumping for joy on the inside, saying *"YES! You see? You're THIN! Now, keep it up."*

It's the emotion, the high, the challenge, and the need to be perfect.

In the end, the eating disorder isn't about the food—it's about the emotions behind it.

In the end, the cancer isn't just the actual disease, but what has manifested on the deepest levels within the mind and the body.

I was sick. I was very, very sick.

> *"Chemo #7! Hopefully, I'll only have one left. My weight was 111 pounds today, with clothes. Rachael [,the nurse,] said she knows I don't like to eat high fats, so I need to increase my protein. I hate talking about food."*

I wrote a lot over the next few weeks. Most of it was related to food, weight, binging and purging. Surprisingly, or maybe not, not much had to do with the actual cancer itself.

Until June 9th:

"I can honestly say I am scared. Today, I had my gallium injection and Wednesday I go for my CT Scan (God! I hate drinking that [barium]!) And then my gallium scan at 9:30am. Early morning. Whether I continue with chemo really depends if the tiny spot on my spleen is from Hodgkin's or something else, such as a cyst or a bruise.

"I am so scared. The only thing I can do is try to rest my nerves...I do not know, and do not want to know, what my reaction will be if I have to do more chemo. My body is deteriorating!"

However, you can't just switch off an eating disorder because cancer makes an appearance in your life. Addictions don't work like that.

"No one's home. There's good food. It's the perfect opportunity [to binge and purge]. Yet, I struggle with the voices in my head and tell myself: Haven't you learned your lesson yet? Wasn't cancer a big enough rock to your head?"

Nope.

Still June:

"Yesterday was like a day from hell. CT Scans, gallium scans, barium, IVs, needles, throwing up. Gross. Need I continue? They didn't use my PICC line for inserting the dye for the CT Scan because the radiologist...told me they would get a better reading (especially of the spleen) if they did it through an IV. It hurt, but at least they got it on the first try! I threw up after the scan because of the barium. I hate that stuff. I do NOT like being forced to drink something I hate (ED)."

So, perhaps it wasn't the barium, it was my fear that there were calories in it? The self awareness I have today that I had yet to learn then.

"Today I had a yogurt, coffee and a big chicken salad with vinegar. It was good. I'm going to drink my [green] tea now and then go to bed soon. I'll add an apple and a yogurt to that list after tea. Total: 550-600 calories. Not enough; but I didn't purge today. It feels good to feel good."

"I need to eat! My pants are falling off! Breathe, Sara, breathe. Take deep breaths! Ahh...now go eat, [Sara] before you lose another pound!"

Don't believe those last words. I acted like I cared, but secretly inside I was ecstatic that I was so thin. It's a game, sometimes in the eating disordered mind, to pretend or to play coy like you are "trying" to gain weight, but the little voice in your head is jumping, celebrating, saying, "YES!" It's a lie. It's a game. It's not real. You're only fooling yourself by lying to anyone, and more than anything, you're lying to your self.

The results from my exams came back, a bit inconclusive, and they still weren't able to determine whether the spot on my spleen was from cancer or previous scarring.

My oncologist ordered more chemotherapy.

I protested.

We got a second opinion.

"The doctors won't have an answer for me until next Thursday when we meet with the adult oncologist at Yale, explained Dr. Cooper. The 'limbo' period from now until Thursday is going to suck."

Thursday:

> *"Bad morning. Left with a lot of tough choices. Chemo, Radiation, meet somewhere in between. Help! Weighed 113.5 lbs with clothes. I don't know how I feel about [my weight]. I like Dr. Cooper. I wish I didn't cry the whole time and actually talked with him. I should thank him for his efforts. PET Scan was completely negative. Good news. Still, I'm not happy. I'm falling apart."*

Late June, we were looking into second opinions, overseas studies, and pretty much anything that would suggest otherwise; anything to forgo additional chemotherapy treatment. I physically felt like I couldn't endure any more chemotherapy. It is designed to kill cells, cancer cells and the good ones, and I already felt dead—on the inside and on the outside. I intuitively feared any additional chemo would send me over the edge, and set me up for graver complications in the future for secondary cancers, additional damage to my organs, or other side effects that come along with these chemicals.

The results from all of the tests:

> *"Still no answers, still no decisions. Nothing. It's 1pm No word from Dr. Cooper. [The pediatric oncologist] said she recommended 'definitely more chemotherapy.' I cried at the thought. I didn't stop crying until half an hour after I got home. Help me!"*

Fortunately, one trial study from Germany suggested an alternative that caught our attention and had our interest—something to consider. Instead of additional chemotherapy, I would transition to a slightly more aggressive form of radiation. In the end, it was up to us, my family, and to me the course of treatment and plan of action that I wanted to take. A big decision for a 19-year old to take on, that would decide her future life, or potential lack there of. No one really talks about it, but there is a possibility you can die from chemotherapy and the harmful effects it comes with.

"It's a new day and I have never been happier. Dr. Cooper called and said from the studies done from Austria/ Germany patients who received 4 courses of chemo (6 treatments of OPPA, 2 with COPP) and then followed by radiation had great results and low recurrences. He then said he would feel very comfortable with me stopping at the 4 courses and going on to low-doses of radiation. Yeah!"

I was in to start the new treatment regime as per Dr. Cooper's suggestion.

I developed a very bad infection within my body, leaving me in excruciating pain. Everything hurt, to the point that I couldn't get out of bed. This was different than the pain I had felt from chemotherapy. Something deadly was attacking me. With a very high fever, I was rushed immediately back to Yale New Haven Hospital for investigation. After a while, you start to feel like a patient number, a disease, and an experiment, with all of the tests they run on you.

"I woke up Friday morning running a fever of 104°F. Went to the hospital and almost fainted while taking X-rays. Blood Pressure was 80/40 (low!). They stuck an IV in me, which restricted every move, [which was attached] to a metal pole, a pump and a bag of liquids. Two nights in a hospital and I was going crazy. God bless those kids who are in there longer."

I was admitted to the hospital as an inpatient for recovery; my parents spent every moment they could with me, bringing me the snacks and foods I liked. I hated being in bed in the hospital, attached to a pole with the IVs dangling from my arm. I felt like a trapped bird in a cage, not free, but tied down, in every way.

With a lack of entertainment, I watched whatever VHS tape (millennials reading this, you may need to Google what a VHS tape is) I could find in the children's inpatient ward. *Maid In Manhattan* was the only movie I could find. To this day, I despise that movie, and Jennifer Lopez as an actress (aside from Selena). Sorry, not sorry, J.Lo.

One night I felt anxious from sitting so long in bed. After eating whatever snacks I had available in my room, and from what I could find in the hospital floor communal kitchen, I ate as much as I could before lulling my sad body, IV-ed arm, and metal pole to the bathroom to throw up. Shameful, to this day, and so sad to reflect on, being that sick in a hospital yet still fixated on this addiction—it was the only way I knew how to cope with all the pain I was feeling.

That's an eating disorder.

One day, we escaped. My parents and I left the hospital, much to the dismay of the hospital staff. We went to eat at Subway to get something other than the terrible hospital food. Veggie sub had the least calories. I picked apart the pieces of vegetables first, eating one by one, then the bread, just like I used to in high school. Sick. Sad. Habits. Addictions.

> *"The PICC line is out, the cause of this whole infection, leading to my overnight stay at the grand 10th floor, East Pavilion, Room 728 suite...I hope I can start radiation soon and my hair will stop falling out and start growing back (it's been four weeks [since my last chemotherapy]!?).*"

While awaiting the start of my radiation treatments, my appetite slightly returned after the grueling chemotherapy treatment, yet the eating disorder continued.

July 2003:

> *"I'm hungry (mentally) and feel like a pig because I'm eating so much. I wish I could eat evenly all day and not eat as much at night. It's okay as long as I don't taste the food the next morning [from overeating at night]. That's the worst for me, and a huge trigger.*
>
> *1 (more) yogurt*
> *3 (more) pieces of bread*
> *1500 calories for today*
>
> *Oink. oink. oink. oink..."*

The first of two radiation phases had started. During this treatment, I felt like an experiment. They line you up with precise measures on a table in a cold room, no shirt on, as they draw little marks with Sharpies to pinpoint exactly where they will treat with radiation. The markings secure that it's the same area each day, and to be sure any remaining cancer cells are killed within you.

Phase 1 targeted my neck, and upper chest area.

What's bizarre is I actually still love the smell of Sharpie markers. There's something about their artistic connotative nature.

End of Journal number 2 concludes:

> *"I wish I could end this journal on a better note; perhaps an 'I'm glad I can look back on all of this because I'm done with this Eating Disorder' [kind of ending]. I hate to say it, but I think I'll still be dealing with it for a while. That doesn't*

mean I have to act on it, I just think that distorted eating disorder voice will remain in my head a little while longer. I'll deal with battling cancer, and I'll deal with battling this eating disorder. In the end, I'll win against both. I'm stronger than the two put together, multiplied by ten."

Checkmate, cancer. Oh the power of the mind.

AUGUST 2003

"Need to write. Need to plan. Need to get over this [cancer and eating disorder] now! Ask the whys, plan ahead, put myself in a good head-space, learn my boundaries, and live a healthy life. The unknown is scary, but it can't be worse than an eating disorder; or, even worse, cancer."

"Today was the last day of my first part of radiation. I have until September 2nd to live free [without treatment until the next phase]."

Yes. I actually wrote those words **LIVE FREE** 12 years before the conception of **Live Free Warrior** and **Living Free.** Sometimes you are who you are before you realize it. The seeds—as mentioned in the opening quote of this chapter—had been blown, but the terrain was not yet ready.

The next three "live free" weeks' journal entries consisted of internal battles and scribbles of binging and purging, fighting off urges, notes of what I ate, and thinking that I needed to go to the gym more. Priorities? An interesting version of living free...

Phase 2 of radiation began, targeting my abdomen and spleen. I remember them covering my uterus and lower abdominal area to protect any potential fertility damage by radiation, in the case I wanted to have children in the future.

I said, *"I don't care. I don't want to have children."*

They said, *"You're 19, you will change your mind."*

I didn't, and I won't. But, I applaud their efforts. Once again, sometimes you know who you are before you realize it.

LAST DAY OF TREATMENT, SEPTEMBER 29, 2003

"Two months until my [20th] birthday. I'm done. Well, I'm done with treatments, that is."

Mind you, at the same time, my mother's father was still battling lung cancer, which has metastasized to his brain. At this point, he was transitioned from the hospital to a care center for his remaining days.

"It was very sad to see my grandfather like he was. I can't imagine how my mom feels. Facing death and seeing it in someone can be emotional and moving, especially because I had cancer, and beat it (knock-on-wood that it never comes back, EVER). However, my grandfather is going to have a lot of work to do in heaven when he's watching over all of us."

OCTOBER 18, 2003, STRATFORD, CT

"My grandfather died on Tuesday. Today is Saturday. He looked a lot more peaceful at his wake than when I would go see him at Lord Chamberlain [care center] gasping for

air. I do love him, and I know he'll be beside God watching over me and my family."

For very few, the answer to living free is death, and the end of the life cycle after too long of a battle.

For the rest of us, the answer is rebirth, to renew, to be reborn, and to learn to **LIVE FREE.**

PART 2

"CANCER" AS A GIFT
(A.D. AFTER CANCER'S DEATH)

↗

"CANCER" AS A GIFT
INTRODUCTION

"Just living is not always living. Look at your life. Can you call it a blessing. Can you call it a gift, a present of existence? Would you like this life to be given to you again and again?"

— *Osho, from What is Courage*

I'm writing this introduction on National Cancer Survivor's Day, June 3, 2018, in the United States. I was clueless about the day, until an email popped up in to my inbox from my mom as a reminder of the day. Her message:

"Good morning Sarita! Love you so much!! Always grateful they cured your cancer. Please always remember that when things seem tough, they were a lot worse 15 years ago. And without your health, you have nothing."

When I read this, I immediately stopped what I was doing, and cried. They were, of course, joyful tears; it was the message I needed to hear in that exact moment. To stop, pause, and remember the "gift" that cancer had given me, and my perspective on life, and why I chose the path towards living free.

I had completely different plans for my day today. The to-do list included emails, follow-up plans for the week ahead, video editing, content planning—pretty much, everything related to work.

However, after receiving this message, I canceled my plans and my original agenda for the day. Instead, I felt compelled more than ever to start this section of the book. Cancer can have that positive long-term side effect as well. It reminds you that, deep within your soul you know that life is precious, and that eventually, we will all die. What we do in the day to day to enjoy it to its fullest, and care for our bodies AND our minds, to live the longest, healthiest lives we possibly can? This is for me, the most important "to-do" on our daily talk list (next to brushing our teeth, that's important too).

Jokes aside, I can't emphasize enough, that true strength and power comes from the mind. It's the only true source that can wake us up, to believe and create desire in a thought or a purpose, and be our own fuel for creating change in our lives. No one else will do it for you.

Awareness. Choice. Action.

Those are the three simplest steps to creating change or transformation. Those three simple, yet challenging steps, all come from the mind. Awareness, choice and action are three powerful steps towards creating a life of living free.

I realized that if anorexia taught me something, it's that the power of the mind can truly overpower anything in the body and the environment around us. Time to put that power to good use, to overcome the demons, the diseases, and, of course, the cancers I was allowing to control my life.

↗

CHAPTER 5:
FINDING PURPOSE + PASSION

"She needs time, like we all do.
Time to be ok with being ok.
Because sometimes feeling right,
after feeling so wrong for so long,
is the hardest thing to get used to."

— *JM Storm*

This Page Left Intentionally Blank.

A blank page. The calm, after the storm. Stillness and silence. What the hell does one do? For months, almost a full year, you have people buzzing, whizzing, flooding and whirring around you. You're on a schedule, being monitored, watched, weighed, poked, and measured down to every beating pulse.

One day, it all just stops. After the storm, what comes next?

For months (for some, years), you have a schedule and agenda of appointments, check-ins, needles, scans, doctors, and flocks of people in scrubs and white jackets buzzing around you.

"So, this is the point in your life when you started practicing yoga, right?" I get asked in interviews this time and time again.

Nope. I still had many more lessons to learn before then. Buckle up. Back to Boston we go.

After finishing my treatments, I had suffered from Post-Traumatic Stress Dis-order (PTSD). This left me in a state of, *"What the hell do I do with my life now?"*

The following years after my last treatment was a series of follow-up treatments that trickled out from monthly, to tri-monthly, to bi-annually, to annual scans and check-ups. In between, life resumed as it was before cancer. Concerns were related to college, my relationship with my boyfriend, and my weight. Life was back to normal, I guess, one could say.

OCTOBER 21, 2003, THREE WEEKS AFTER MY FINAL RADIATION TREATMENT

"Things are OK lately. I feel pressured, stressed and

overwhelmed by school. I feel unaccomplished too, like I should be doing more with my life and [be] more goal-oriented. I feel like I teeter every day about what job I want to have and that I should be doing something, other than school, right now to get [myself] there...I'm in no rush to be a fully responsible adult (I need to have some fun in these college years!), but I feel like a nobody a lot...[and] school feels so juvenile and unimportant."

Finishing college, however, was my ticket out. I was ready, when given the chance, to take that ticket and go have some fun.

In the two months that followed my last treatment, interestingly enough, I didn't note a word about cancer in my journal. My notes were fully focused on what I was eating, what I was trying not to throw up, who was pissing me off, what I was going to do with my life, and my weight.

NOVEMBER 19, 2003

"Got weighed at the hospital on Monday—49.6 kilos, 109 lbs... with clothes...no comment."

Don't believe it. I was thrilled. I loved the feeling of my bones, the physical trophy of triumph over the need for food and the control I had over my own body once again.

Your eating disorder friend? She's a big, stinky little liar. She sucks, and will tell you things that aren't true just to keep her around. And, if you're not ready to deal with her antics, she has a big brother who will take her place. His name?

Alcoholism.

SEPTEMBER 2004, COLLEGE: TAKE 2

The following fall, I enrolled in undergrad at Suffolk University, and later the New England School of Art & Design (NESAD) in Boston, Massachusetts. Learning from my last experience at college, I didn't even consider staying in the dorms this time. I had a centrally located private studio apartment right on the corner of the Boston Commons.

It also conveniently happened to be one block away from a CVS (binge and purge materials), a liquor store, and an alley full of clubs and bars.

My boyfriend, Pat, did not move up to Boston this time around and we attempted a long-distance relationship between Connecticut and the city. He came up a few weekends in the beginning, we had fun, drinking and partying, like back in the day the first time we came up to Boston together.

We could feel the space, the distance and the completely different lifestyle (I was away at college and he was back at home working in CT) building between us. We had been together just under five years at that point, going through things that not many couples at that age experience. I was a free bird at last, living on my own, and we were changing as people.

One night, shortly after one of what would be his last visits up to Boston to see me, I went out with one of my guy friends (guys were always easier to hang out with, even in high school, for me—less drama?). We all drank a lot, and the next morning I woke up in bed with one of the roommates who I had been attracted to, realizing we had slept together.

I called Pat the next day and said we needed to break up, and that I needed my space to be on my own, and not in a relationship. I honestly don't remember if I told him exactly what had happened, but either way, I was not proud, and knew no one deserved to be cheated on or dragged through anymore of my debauchery and get hurt in the process.

This time in my life was certainly not my brightest, shining, or clearest moments. Many nights I blacked out, lost count of how many drinks I had, and spent too many mornings trying to recollect the previous nights' events.

I was thin, but not as underweight as I had been after chemotherapy. Determined to do better in school, complete my classes and assignments, and become the straight-A student once again, as I had always in the past, I was determined to make it happen. I would drink, throw up, be a scholar, and prove I could do it all.

I miraculously did do it all. It's not a proud moment, and I honestly don't know how I was able to pull off making all of my classes, assignments, tests, finals, and school projects with the amount of alcohol I was consuming on (at one point) a daily basis.

I wore a drink like a fashion statement in my hand, dancing on the club floor, a jack and diet coke with a swizzle stick (and don't waste any room on the ice) like it was the new black. When I was at home—alone—vodka shots with a chaser of Fresca or crystal light (zero calories) was my drink of choice.

It's terrible, to think back on those times, wondering how much more I could have gotten out of school and from those classes, had I had a clearer, less buzzed mind. To this day, I love learning new things, and as much as I wanted to be grown-up and in the real world already as an adult, I deep down always wanted to be a student, learning new things, for life.

Here's when I tried my first yoga class—and it wasn't love at first downward-facing dog. At the time, I was working part-time at a gym in Boston for the free membership. The college gym just wasn't doing it for me. I needed a place that was clean, professional, and free of college noise, somewhere I could workout and burn some calories. At that time, I preferred my typical gym workout of weights and cardio machines; I hadn't yet embraced the breathing and moving of a yoga flow. I recall taking my first yoga class—a Power Yoga class—at age 21. It was some gym version of an ashtanga flow. I walked out after the nap (savasana), and hopped right on to an elliptical machine to get my "real workout in."

My first yoga class didn't win me over, and it wasn't until four years later that I really started to connect with yoga. After one or two classes at the gym "trying" to like yoga, I stopped wasting my precious gym time and went back to the cardio and weights—plus, I could track how many calories I was burning that way.

Fast forward through the first two years of college, because it's a lot of the same, a buzzed, blurred mix of events. Below are a few highlights to note from the college reel:

- I enrolled in the communications and journalism college department with a major in advertising and double minor in Spanish and graphic design (I later dropped the Spanish minor).

- I was hospitalized not once, not twice, but three times for alcohol intoxication.

- Miraculously, I never woke up in some random person's bed, but always safely (albeit hung over) in my own.

- Equally miraculous, I never lost my wallet or passport in any bar, club, or on the dance floor, no matter how drunk I was.

- Career choice was decided, I would be a Creative Director in an agency.

- I fell in love with art school, and loved my time spent there drawing, crafting, creating, painting, and designing.

- I moved from downtown Boston to the North End waterfront to a charming 2 bedroom, 1 bath I shared with a roommate—my first roommate since the initial attempt at college.

- My junior year, I was invited to a party at a club called The Liquor Store one block away from me in that alley laden with clubs and bars. It was someone's kid brother's 21st birthday party. I loved any excuse to acceptably, socially drink, so, of course joined the festivities. I rode the mechanic bull they had there for 27 seconds that night. I was incredibly thin at the time. And, I met the birthday boy, a young Italian man named Marco.

- The summer before my senior year of college, I had the opportunity to either intern at a business in Boston, return back to Connecticut for the break (wasn't even an option in my mind), or study abroad with a design group in Italy. I chose Italy. It was a magical 6 weeks living, painting, studying art history and enjoying some of the best espressos of my life in the streets, hillsides and cafes of Florence, Rome and Venice. I drank way too much during the evenings, being alone, living with three other girls, and nowhere to binge and purge. So, alcohol was an easier method to use to cope with my confused emotions.

- Coming back from Italy, the World Cup was in the final match. Italy won against France in a tied 1-1 match, 5-3 penalty shot in overtime. Living in the North End, the little Italy of Boston, we celebrated all day long. I drank...all day long. I also ran into the Italian Stallion (Marco) in the evening on Hanover Street.

• In a drunken blur, one night I decided to pick up my watercolors again and started painting. It was an Italian flag, but messy, in the way the Pirates of the Caribbean font looks, on screen. Over it was my last initial, a Q. Shortly after that, I got my first tattoo on my inner left wrist. I felt like an Italian badass.

Marco and I began dating shortly after in September of 2006. He had (has) one of the kindest hearts and most forgiving souls. He gave me that secure feeling that life would simply be just fine by his side. I was never a princess kind of girl, but at that point in my life, I needed a bit of a rescue. That, or my drunk-ass would have fallen down the wrong stairs, lost a shoe in Faneuil Hall or woke up on a Boston Commons park bench in the middle of November. It's freezing in Boston that time of year.

We dated, we danced, we partied, and we fell in love. I was the life of the party, spending Friday and Saturday nights dancing in Boston bars until last call at 1am. Sunday afternoons, if I was alone, were spent staving off a hangover by continuing to drink until the next morning. Numbing out emotions, and a hangover, at the same time.

There's a point, however, where the life of the party becomes a noticeable problem. Fortunately, i wasn't the angry kind of drunk that punched doors in and got into bar fights, but rather the dance all night, drink too much, black out and sometimes piss the bed kind of drunk.

Neither is good, and both are a problem. However, when you're an alcoholic, it's not that easy to see the problem from the same point of view of others around you.

I got Shingles, which is the adult version of chicken pox. They're painful, can be disgusting looking, and can be caused (like any illness) from a suppressed immune system. The band of nerve-damaging pink, scaly spots wrapped around my torso like a hook, from my right breast all the way to the spinal column. Given medications to heal, I had to stop drinking. And I did, for 21 days.

After the Shingles went away, the partying continued. One late Spring Saturday afternoon, after a blurry night of partying, Marco and I went to a nearby beach about 40 minutes outside of the city. Sitting on the sand together, reflecting no the night before, I remember him saying, *"You know you have to stop at some point. Right, Bella?"*

I knew it. At that point it was clear: I was no longer viewed as the life of the party, but viewed as the girl with a problem.

Being with Marco, who was incredibly family-oriented, 100% Italian, who lived with his immediate family, his cousins and "zios" (aunts and uncles) next door, they became the family and grounding that I didn't have living on my own in Boston. We were incredibly different, but being around Marco and his family reminded me that "fun" and "self-love" don't have to come in the form of partying. And being around an Italian family, I was forced to see that food was an incredibly joyful experience for many people who aren't struggling with an eating disorder.

Around the same time, I graduated high honors from Suffolk University/ NESAD with a BFA in Advertising and Graphic Design. I was ready to take on the adult world, but in a very undeveloped and confused mind and body.

EARLY SUMMER 2007

Here's the light. This was the "aha" moment. This was the point in my life that I decided enough was enough and I wanted to create a better life for myself. No one pushed me, this time. This came from a purely intuitive voice that was guiding me to take charge, stop being a victim of the "cancers" I was allowing into my life, If I truly wanted to "control" my life, then I had to take responsibility for my actions, before anything.

I saw a future in my life, a future I wanted to create and make better for myself. I suddenly wanted to get married someday, and create something more than a series of blurry mornings and forgotten nights. A light went off inside me, and I followed it.

I quit drinking. Just like that. I know it doesn't work like that for most people. However, that's how I stopped. There was no more partying three nights a week and no more drinking, I now spent my time at Marco's family's house, applying for jobs in creative departments around the city, and using bulimia once again to dull and numb my new emotions.

The thing with addictions is, they don't just go away. For me, I simply swapped one for the other. When I wasn't drinking, I was throwing up, and when I wasn't throwing up, I was drinking. Whatever it is you're avoiding and don't want to feel, it needs a drug, vice, or addiction to free it, or (better said) forget it. However, they don't get resolved with that strategy.

JULY 2007, BOSTON, MA

I went back to Connecticut for an annual exam at the hospital, as part of my post-cancer follow-up care. The general care letter from the oncologist to my pediatrician kept in content reads:

June 21, 2007

"Dear Dr. [Pediatrician],

"Sara was seen in our clinic today. She is now almost four years from completion of therapy for Hodgkin's disease. She has just graduated from Boston University [no I didn't—it was Suffolk University/NESAD, thank you], Magna Cum Laude and looking for a job in marketing. Sara reports she has been doing well...

"Although Sara appeared well, her weight is very concerning to us, at a mere 47 kg. Sara reports that she is eating well, but did not elaborate on what that encompasses. We were able to speak with her mother, who reports that although Sara's weight is down, she is not concerned. She has watched her eat full meals and snacks while with her. Often since her anorexia was diagnosed, during times of change and stress her weight will drop but then recover to baseline.

"Today, Sara's exam was remarkable for her emaciated appearance...PET/CT showed no evidence of disease..."

It's funny how appearances can be easily created or falsified. I was very underweight at the time, both limiting my food intake, working out in excess, and purging in an effort to keep my weight down.

Around this time, I landed my first job as a Junior Art Director at Hill Holliday Advertising Agency. If you are at all familiar with the ad world, this is a BFD, or Big Fucking Deal, to land a position like that just out of college. I was thrilled, and more motivated than ever to straighten my ass out and be a functioning human contributing to society in a healthier, more creative way.

The job was fantastic, and I loved the energy of working there. It was a dream, really, and I felt blessed to have the opportunity.

After a bit of convincing, I sold Marco on the idea to get matching tattoos on the inside of our left wrists. It was a logo I had designed, combing both of our last name initials: a Q and a G. After all I had been through (up to this point) in my life, I felt s strong attachment to my last name Quiriconi and this tattoo was a visual "promise" to each other of a future together.

The next year, Marco and I decided to move in together. The middle ground for him moving outside of his family's home was a condo complex about 10 minutes away from their house. I moved out of the city, and into the suburbs of Dedham, Massachusetts.

In truth, I loved him, but hated living there. I have always loved the vibe and energy of cities. In the 'burbs, it was quiet, lonely, and disconnecting, for me.

There was a new development in the works a short walk from where we lived. Behind a Costco, there were building Legacy Place, which had a Whole Foods, and L.L. Bean, some other chain stores, and a yoga studio in the works.

I was commuting in and out of the city to work via the train, where I felt oddly left out of the mix of adults who had office attire, pencil skirts, rolled up socks and sneakers, which were much more comfortable, I'd assume, than heels for the trek in to the city. I liked commuting for about a month. Then, it got old. I missed the city life, and dreamed of being back there. However, I chose something different to create a life with Marco, and it was a decision I had to deal with at the time.

DECEMBER 2008, BOSTON, MA

On December 22nd we got engaged. It was a very creative proposal, on Marco's part, counting the days we had been together, tricking me in to thinking I was going to a basketball game, which turned in to be a walk through the North End where we had first met and fallen in love. It was beautiful. We were surrounded by the buzz of the city, yet the silence of the snow.

The engagement ring was exactly as I had wanted: a 1-Karat princess cut diamond with a platinum band. I had picked it out, as I didn't want any surprises; I thought this ring was what would make our marriage happy. It would be a symbol of our connection.

I was ready to be a wife, and start creating what I thought I "should" be doing as any other woman in her 20's has to do. The checklist was created, and now being achieved:

☒ Graduate from college.

☒ Get a job.

☒ Engagement ring.

☒ Get married (in progress).

☒ Buy a home.

☐ Have kids.

☐ Have the family over for a Thanksgiving meal prepared by me.

☐ Get a dog, or a pet, of some sort (just not a cat...I don't like cats).

☐ Take a family vacation once a year for holidays (with the kids, of course).

☐ Live happily ever after.

That last one is a tall order, I'm aware. But, in my head, checking off the previous boxes would equate to the ultimate goal of happiness. That's what I was told, and that's what I believed.

We all may have our differences in the world, but in the end, we all want health, love and happiness, at its most basic level. It's in our DNA and engrained in us to seek out life experiences that will provide those. Some of us, maybe most of us, just get a little lost in the fulfillment process.

That was the list society had engrained in my mind about what I thought would make me a happy, successful person. I had no clue of what I actually wanted in my life, I didn't know what really made me happy, creative, passionate, and fulfilled; hence, I looked to what society offered up as the standard thinking that would fulfill and fuel me.

However, when you don't know what truly makes you happy and are self-aware, your happiness becomes dependent on that checklist. When one of those "checks" disappears, your sense of happiness, sense of self, and your sense of purpose also disappear. You become dependent, and you become fixated on expectations.

"I am a Junior Art Director at... I am the wife of... I am, I am, I am." Think of a conversation you had recently with someone you just met. I bet, one of the first questions asked was, "So, what do you do?" When we lack a sense of self-awareness and self, we attach to labels and what we grasp on to what define us. It's a recipe for disaster, because a job is never permanent, no matter how high, or low, in the ranks we are.

Work slowed down, and the economy was hit hard. After a second round of layoffs at Hill Holliday, I was a part of the next slaughter. I remember taking the train home the day I was laid-off. I had a small box of my belongings, was in tears crying, calling my parents and feeling devastated. Once again, something I loved was taken away from me, and I was left feeling lost, without an identity, without a job, and with a lot of time on my hands, to cry, to think, and to binge and purge.

It was a tough year of applying to the black hole of inboxes and applications that were never answered or had an auto-reply of *"Thank you for your application. If you're a good fit for our company, we'll kindly get back to you in a timely manner."*

I never heard back. It began to be very clear to me that I wasn't a good fit, and that I wasn't really good at anything anymore. I became incredibly depressed, a royal pain in the ass for Marco, and relied heavily on bulimia to cope and deal with my alone time.

I felt like I failed. Once again, I failed, and I wasn't good enough. Just like I wasn't good enough in high school, I wasn't good enough now to land a job. I followed all the steps I thought I had to do to get me there, but it still wasn't enough to keep the job.

What the fuck?

My saving grace for feeling part of something again was the commuting back and forth to downtown via the train to go to the gym I still had a monthly membership at. It made me feel a part of something with others, instead of the long nine-hour days alone sitting in our apartment in the suburbs looking up the same websites of job listings filled with endless hope. Getting your measly unemployment check in the mail is the saddest reminder that you have fallen below the line that defines success.

On the one hand, you are thankful to have that money, because you probably (like I did) really need it. On the other hand, it is probably only a small portion of what you were making before while working at your full-time job. More importantly, for me, at least, it didn't supply the culture of people around me, nor the title attached to my position.

Unemployment is just about as sexy sounding as bulimia in the eyes of society. Double gross. Double failure. I suck. Fuck my life.

Thankfully, during this time, Marco still had his very secure full-time job as an electrical contractor at a construction company outside the city. This kept us afloat as a couple, and still on track for getting married in a year.

An increase in train fares in Boston, combined with a monthly gym membership, and the lack of unemployment funds meant it became very difficult for me to keep commuting daily in to the city just to get out of the house and go to the gym I loved being a part of. I was losing my connection to the city.

What else could I do for burning calories and movement? I needed something else to keep me active. I got an invite to take a free yoga class at a new studio opening around the corner that was located in that complex I had mentioned, Legacy Place.

Yoga. Hm. How many calories can a yoga class burn? Probably not many, but maybe I can eat a bit less then.

Disconnected, lost, lonely, and depressed, I walked in to Stil Studio in Dedham for the first time and decided to give this "yoga" thing a try.

What happened next will blow you away.

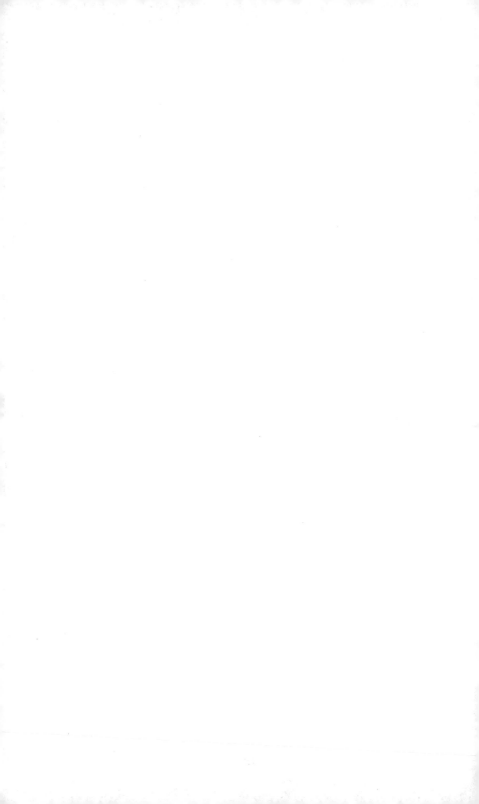

↗

CHAPTER 6:
THE MIND/BODY CONNECTION

"It is part of the cure to wish to be cured."

— *Seneca*

AUGUST 2009, DEDHAM, MASSACHUSETTS

Well, actually, not really. Finding yoga initially didn't blow me away either, but it was a great way to burn some calories and get a workout in.

As I mentioned, I had taken a few yoga classes at the gym I worked at in the past, but nothing ever really clicked for me.

But something was different when I practiced yoga at this studio, and with this particular teacher. It was a different experience for me than any other class or fitness activity I had experienced in the past. Maybe it was my mindset, or my desperation to feel some sort of connection. I honestly believe it was a combination of all of the above.

This yoga, this class—it felt good. And, for the first time in a long time I actually *felt* my body. Not in the way that you pretend to give yourself a hug, or palpate your arm to *feel* the bones or pull at the fat, as I had in the past. This time I could actually feel my body awakening and coming alive. It was like when you decorate your house with Christmas lights, lining all of the windows, the framework, the handrails and mailbox, and then the moment you plug the lights into the socket and see the entire house lit up, you smile and stand back in awe of the beauty before you.

For the first time in a very long eating-disordered journey, I didn't think about how many calories I burned, or if I needed to eat a little less later in the day. For the first time in a long time, I felt good, and I felt *free.*

That's how my body felt: alive, illuminated, awakened, and connected.

After the remainder of my monthly gym membership and commuter rail pass ran out, I signed up for the monthly, unlimited yoga class pass that Stil Studio offered its new community. I was hooked, and gradually took more and more classes, until I was going daily.

Initially, yoga's sole purpose in my life was to make it easier to get in a workout at half of the price I was paying to commute in to the city to go my gym. Even though I had this inner "light" that went off, I was in it for the sweat and the burn.

Keeping up with my new workout regime, I finally got a freelance production job. It was at a women's clothing company in their creative department after a year of applying anywhere. It was a job; however, it was not ideal. The position was very part-time, and it was clear from the beginning they did not want to hire me full-time for the designer position they had open. Plus, the office was outside the city in a tacky, grey, brick building that would have been better suited for a law office than the creative department of a clothing company.

Feeling incredibly left out in many ways, I, once again, got the feeling that I wasn't good enough to make it, nor to be a part of the team. The last dagger to the gut: it was a company, and creative department, of almost all women—clique-y and full of attitude and drama.

It was high school drama, take two.

I despised working there, and yearned for something different. While I learned a lot working in catalog, retail merchandising, and design, I couldn't stand being part of that particular work culture. It was so different than the fun, free vibes of working at the advertising agency. In many ways, I felt like I didn't deserve the better life, and this was what I was stuck with.

We bought our first home together in April 2010. It was a top floor two-bedroom, one-bath, newly remodeled apartment in a multi-family home in Jamaica Plain, Massachusetts. The home was truly beautiful, and I loved the feeling of owning something that was ours to create, design, and make a home out of.

MAY 30, 2010, MASSACHUSETTS

Marco and I got married as planned on Memorial Day weekend of 2010. It was a very traditional wedding, with a bridal party, ivory white dress, ceremony in a church with vows that were scripted (which I was very against, but there's no arguing with a Priest in a Catholic church), and a 150+ reception party on the beach to follow.

Traditional as it was, I refused to a wear a veil, to toss the bouquet, to have big bows placed on the reception chairs, and fought against anything I could rationalize to have a non-traditional wedding. Weeks before the actual wedding day, my mother-in-law at the time said, *"you can't cut your hair short before the wedding!"*

Like hell I can't. I chopped it short like a Posh Spice bob with pride and defiance a few weeks before the big day.

I'm not sure what triggered it, but on our wedding night, I got incredibly drunk. I hadn't drunk alcohol, to that extent since my college days. It was the worse hangover I had felt in a long time. I was throwing up for the first two hours of my official first day of being a wife, and barely made it out to the tables to say thank you and good morning to the guests that had stayed over the night at the hotel.

Maybe it was intuition, that this style of wedding, nor the path I was on, was truly what I wanted. Perhaps it was part of my subconscious plan that I didn't want to remember some part of what I was really committing to.

We can tell ourselves lies, to fit in to what societal standards expect from us. However, when we aren't able to express our honest desires from a stance of self-awareness and intuitive truth, it's easier to turn to the external world for guidance and answers. In the end, something doesn't feel right, and hearts get broken in the process—including marriages.

If I wasn't going to have the wedding I wanted, I was damn sure I would have the ultimate honeymoon. I've always loved traveling. There's something so magical about being in an airport, ready to take off, the excitement of *"where to next."* It's a buzzing feeling of excitement for me, to take off from one place and land in another—a place that can be completely different from your home base.

Athens, Greece, Venice, Italy, the Greek Isles, and Paris, France. Travel transforms you, in many ways for the better.

In addition to rebelling against the traditional wedding, I also rebelled against having to change my last name. I was so attached to Quiriconi, and after the former identities I felt I had parted with in the past, particularly my job title, it killed me to take Marco's last name over mine. For Marco, however, it was important that I did, because that was "tradition," as my family told me: so, I succumbed, settled, and changed it from a Q to a G.

Two weeks later I was in a tattoo shop down the street from our home getting a turtle inked on my lower right hip signifying an S and a Q, in honor of my newly lost last name.

Back in Boston, or, more specifically, the 'burbs, there is nothing more suffocating than a "free bird" feeling captive in a cage. I wanted out. I was done with the production job that I felt over-qualified and under-appreciated for. I cut back from part-time, to very part-time, to the point where I was so part-time they called me in to a corner office to have a "chat."

The two co-creative directors of the catalog department in a kind, yet removed, way told me that they just didn't see the need for my help or services on their upcoming schedule of projects. They thanked me for my time and contributions, and wished me all the best.

I know bullshit when I smell it. I'd appreciate honesty over falsity to save conflict and face. While it hurt to be let go again, at the same time I felt this giant weight being lifted from my shoulders.

I was free and unemployed, once again. A series of conflicting emotions ensued, but it was my reality.

Still practicing yoga, now daily with all of the extra time on my hands, I continued applying to jobs that caught my eye.

An ad called out to me for a freelance designer in downtown working in the creative marketing team for a well-known tee shirt company based in Boston. The awful women's clothing company freelance gig had paid off, and given me the experience I needed to apply, and eventually land, the job as a designer on the team at *Life is good.* Their company motto was *"Do what you love. Love what you do."*

I was offered a full-time job after my interviews, which, after two years of seeking full-time employment as a designer, of course I said YES! and jumped at the opportunity.

I learned a lot working with this company, and from my boss who was a senior designer on the team. She had a keen eye for detail, and a passion for design that was inspiring in many ways. For a while, life at *Life is good* was really good.

Stil Studio was starting a yoga teacher training. I never really wanted to be a teacher, but I was eager to learn more about this practice that was slowly transforming my life. I was eating much better, especially now that I was working full-time. That meant little time alone at home, which was always a huge trigger for me, and now I was useful, part of a team, and with purpose working at *Life is good.*

I signed up for the yoga teacher training, scheduled the Fridays off in advance for the three-day intensive modules booked, and was ready to be a student again. I slowly transformed my work wardrobe from wearing jeans and flats to long black yoga pants and tall black boots that I could easily zip off during the workday to sit cross-legged in my chair.

During one of the busiest parts of the season, designing the new fall catalog, my boss turned to me and said,"You're not going to leave me to become a yoga teacher, right?"

I honestly answered, "No way!" and laughed it off and went back to my work.

The question stuck with me, however, and over time, as the training progressed, the idea didn't sound so crazy.

How I was living my life, working long hours behind a computer, leaving with no energy, creatively drained from outputting my efforts, and in small working quarters with lack of space, doing repetitive work...it was completely the opposite of the new, healthier lifestyle I was learning about and experiencing with yoga.

I liked what I was doing as a designer at *Life is good*, but I didn't LOVE what I was doing. For two years I struggled to find a full-time position working as a designer, back in the city. I had found it, I got it—so, why wasn't I happy?

DECEMBER 2011, BOSTON, MA

I finished my teacher training, eager to share with other students and the world the joy, transformation and change I had experienced by taking on the practice of yoga.

During the graduation party at our teacher training, my teacher offered each one of us a mala with one word signifying our personality or character strength. My word was *determination*. Ironically, it's also the tattoo that I later got on the inside of my upper right arm, where the PICC line had been. This teacher was unbelievable, intuitively smart, and incremental in my transformational process. He was on to something.

After eight months of full-time employment at *Life is good*, I started crafting an exit strategy. I would leave full-time designing and become a full-time yoga teacher.

It was a gradual transition, as I would recommend to anyone looking to change fields of such drastic degrees and pay. Teaching yoga classes did not, and does not, pay that much, and it certainly didn't pay anywhere near what I was making on a weekly basis working at *Life is good*. Nor did it come with any of the paid vacations or health benefits. #entreprenuerlife

Marco supported me during my entire transition to teaching, and was actually one of the driving forces that kept me pursuing this path of teaching. It was a struggle to find classes, clients, and studios to teach at, and often times, harder than it was looking for design jobs. At least there were more agencies and companies needing design than there were studios needing teachers.

My boss wasn't as happy, as one would expect. She was losing a valued team member that she had done a plausible job of teaching and training in the art of photoshop and production editing. I kindly received full support and best wishes from everyone in the Life is good company, including the founders, which was the first time I was leaving something on my own terms, and starting making decisions with my best interest at heart.

My gradual plan to transition from design to teaching was working at an athletic clothing store with strong ties to community while seeking teaching jobs to slowly take over my schedule. This clothing store offered its employees the opportunity to take classes for free on a weekly basis, which was a great way to network while looking for classes in local studios.

Working retail for your family's business (the ski shop) and working retail for a corporate chain company are two very different experiences.

Living under someone else's rules, authority, strict guidelines while being the upbeat, happy, vibrant floor team, pretending to be super excited about the latest stretchy pants that just arrived on the floor... it simply was not me. While I liked the clothing, I hated drinking the kool-aid.

Something important that this company did was to inspire me to later create the **Live Free Manifesto**, which I'll go in to greater detail in the last and final chapter of this book.

I wanted out. And, once again, that's exactly what I did. I was learning to be happy, and making decisions that were based on feeling, truth, honesty, and intuition. There are always choices to be made in life—we just need the courage, the intelligence, planning and time to make them.

Leap, and the net will appear. Eventually, it did. I was teaching yoga full-time in Boston and enjoying every minute of it. I went from teaching two classes a week at a small start-up gym studio and blossomed to a full schedule of 13 classes a week. It wasn't the highest number of classes I have taught in a week, nor the most money I've ever earned; however, in that time, for me, it was enough to be proud of and feel successful in my new career path.

It's important to share, at this point of discovery I wasn't binging and purging, nor drinking. I still didn't have a great relationship or appreciation for my body, but I wasn't active in my previous vices and harmful habits. My weight remained fairly steady at this time, ebbing and flowing five or so pounds based on the season of active summers and cold winters.

Now an official yoga teacher, I ate up the words of Sanskrit and enjoyed learning a new language. I adore learning languages and dialects. It's one of the easiest ways, I find, to connect and understand a culture and connect with its people and meaning—especially when traveling!

One of my favorite words I discovered in Sanskrit was "sankalpa" that loosely translates to determination, purpose or will. When I heard that definition, I knew I had found my next tattoo. Based on signs of the past, such as my will to change my life, the *determination* title my teacher had given me, and the newfound *purpose* in my life, this was IT.

I had the tattoo placed on the inner, upper right arm where the PICC line had been placed during my chemotherapy. The line had connected directly to my heart, and getting the tattoo here signified and reminded me to stay true to my purpose and passions that stem from the heart. In doing so, combined with determination and will to push through the challenging moments, I will remain happy and fulfilled.

FEBRUARY 2013, MIAMI BEACH

Stil Studio was leading a yoga teacher's retreat in Miami Beach, Florida. I have always loved the warm weather, and this retreat sounded like a great excuse to get the hell out of the New England cold and soak in some sun doing what I loved.

I fell in love with Miami. It was February and I didn't need seven layers of bundling up to go outside. Why the hell did I stay in the cold weather for all of these years if there were other places to move to and live?

The seed was planted.

SUMMER 2013, BOSTON, MA

Back to Boston, and back to that checklist, it seemed like a good time to try having a baby. Why not? It's the natural next step, we already had a home, and many other friends around us were pregnant or talking about trying to get pregnant. In a way, it's contageous: when one person does it, it seems like so many others around catch the bug and pop up with baby bumps.

Remember, I didn't want to have children in the past. However, I also wasn't really interested in getting married at that time when I was in my early twenties either. The same voice that created that checklist over-rode my instincts, and rebooted them become "maternal" instincts.

We tried. Nothing happened.

After years of destroying my body, having irregular periods, throwing up, starving, drinking, and self-hatred, my body didn't know how to function in a traditional pro-creative way. My period was still fairly irregular, and after years of being on the pill, it would takes months to wean off of it and give my body the chance to operate on its own again.

We tried for six more months. Nothing happened.

I spent a lot of time in downward facing dog with all of the yoga I was practicing and teaching. Staring back at my feet, seeing the high arches of my grounding and base, I had discovered my next tattoo: *ancora imparo*, Italian for *"Always learning."* It was a phrase Michelangelo had on the inside of a bracelet when he we paint the Sistine Chapel—inverted. Hm. So was a downward-facing dog?

For me, this represented that any time life was turned upside-down there was always something to learn from it. Even when it appears you are fucked up, you can restart, reground and come back to home base at downward-facing dog.

OCTOBER 2013, MIAMI BEACH

I was obsessed with movement and yoga at this time (still am) in my life. When I was introduced to the practice of Budokon®Yoga, I knew I had to find out more about this style of practice. It was strong, which I liked, and masculine, yet feminine at the same time. It had "warrior" energy written all over it, balancing strength and effort, with beauty and grace.

I signed up for the next training for Budokon Yoga, which was being offered at the same hotel and center where my previous yoga teacher retreat was held. It appeared meant to be.

Both Marco and I flew down together this time. During the very long days of my trainings, he enjoyed the relaxed vibes of Miami and explored the beaches and streets of South Beach. We both loved the area, and started to wonder if we could create a life, a family, and make a living there.

During the training, I had a conversation with one of the fellow trainees in between a practice session. He asked me, *"Is it ever hard being with someone who does something completely opposite of you?"*

My answer was short, thoughtless, and a bit defensive on Marco's part, saying, *"Nah. He always supports me in what I'm doing. It's fine that way."*

Was it?

The last evening of the training, I went back to the Airbnb we were staying at for the week and I told Marco I didn't want to have a kid and wanted to stop trying—immediately. He had no clue of what had happened, exactly. This man, who is 100% Italian, and literally has the blood born within him to be a father figure, was of course hurt and taken aback. However, he knew having a baby is not something you push on someone with lightness.

We stopped trying, and I went back on birth control. Still, I wanted to take care of "something" in my life. Maybe it wasn't a baby. But I still had this yearning inside me to nurture something other than a dying plant in the corner of our home.

NOVEMBER 2013, BOSTON, MA

One month later, after much begging, pleading, convincing, and coaxing, we were driving west of the city to pick up the most adorable, perfect looking, and heart-warming puggle name Mary Kate.

Mary Kate? All I could think of was the Olsen twin. That wouldn't do. "Pepino" (Spanish for cucumber) was one of my favorite words I saw at the grocery store during a trip to Puerto Rico. It was a joke at the time, but I did mention if we ever got a pet, I would name him Pepino. Well, Mary Kate was a girl, so we feminized the masculine word and the 12-week old Pepina the Puggle was welcomed in to our lives.

I hadn't had a dog since I was a very young kid. I clearly forgot how much work they were to take care of as pups. If this was what it was like to take care of a puppy, then I was so glad with my decision to not have a kid.

Our marriage at the time was far from perfect. Clearly a child, nor a puppy, would fix what was broken. Pepina was a beautiful distraction and really added so much joy back in to our deteriorating love for one another. However, as we would soon come to realize, adding another element in to the relationshp won't fix what may be already breaking, or already broken.

It was clear our differences in family values and goals were conflicting and causing stress. We tried therapy, to attempt working on our strained relationship. After the fifth or so session, the therapist stopped listening, looked at both of us and said, "Wow. You two really are different."

Thank you so much for having us pay you to tell us that. That was the last therapy session we went to with her.

Winter passed. It would be the last one we would spend in Boston. For the next eight months, I (once again) begged, sold, convinced, and pleaded with Marco to move to Miami. This was our last attempt to see if a change in environment, a new start, and a new home could offer us a new beginning to work through our tears. We really did care about one another. Before anything, we were good friends, and then partners. Perhaps a change of scenery could help?

¡Vamos a Miami!

SEPTEMBER 2014, MIAMI, FLORIDA

We never even visited or saw the apartment we moved to, but on September 6th, Pepina and I flew down from New York City to Miami to meet Marco, who was driving with our U-Haul full packed up with our life in boxes.

What I didn't pack in that U-Haul? Ironic maybe, or perhaps intuition... I didn't take any of our wedding photos, albums, items or memories.

In our new home, our new neighborhood, and with a fresh start for us all, it was time to officiate the *"Live Free"* as a tattoo. Near and dear to my heart, I had the hand-written words inked on my left ribs in a parlor just west of the city.

Live Free Warrior was coming to LIFE.

Four months later, in late winter, after a screaming match of a fight, we both sat there defeated on the bed. Me in tears, as he looked at me and finally allowed the words that I had been trying to tell him for months now, to leave his mouth:

"This isn't going to work, is it."

"No. I said. It isn't."

While the marriage couldn't be saved, thankfully, the friendship has been. Marco and I remain very supportive and friendly with one another, both still living in the same city, with pup-custody visits anytime I want to see my little girl, Pepina.

The following month I moved out of the apartment. I was living on the beach, teaching yoga full time, mixing classes with small group classes, private clients, events and retreats. I was making enough to get by, and even though I was alone, I felt that urge of freedom, independence and LIVE FREE once again.

SUMMER 2015, MIAMI BEACH, FLORIDA

Living on my own offered the freedom that I so yearned for when we were married. It wasn't necessarily being married that I felt tied down from, but the lack of me being who I truly was and needed to be to thrive in the relationship we had. We were different people, and at our cores, we weren't going to change.

Living in a new state and city also offered me the opportunity to have a fresh start and gave me a clean slate to be whoever I really wanted to be.

Something that didn't change? How I coped with stress when I was on my own. I relied heavily on bulimia once again, as a way to manage the stress and anxiety I was feeling of being by myself and alone, feeling lost once again.

I taught a lot of classes during this time. It was a way to keep my mind occupied, and it was a necessary means to make money. For the first time in a very long time, I was on my own again. There was no rent to split, no husband to cover health insurance. It was me myself and I to fend for it all. It's scary as a woman, and it's certainly scarier on a yoga teacher salary.

My parents, of course, had their concerns, and as always let me know they were there to support me in any way I needed. Stubborn mule and determined Sara always knew this in the back of her mind, but I also felt the need to do it on my own and prove that I could. It's part of the challenge I put on myself. I'm my toughest critic when it comes to anything, from sports, to creative projects (ahem, this book!), to my looks. This is a cancer, it's an eating disorder, it's an addiction, and it's a stressful way to live.

I dealt with it all, on my own, through bulimia.

Drinking and teaching yoga definitely wasn't going to happen. Your private client paying $100+ an hour for a session would have every right to be pissed and not pay for the session if you showed up hungover or smelling like vodka. But bulimia? No one would really notice if you were throwing up the night before and didn't eat the next morning.

That's the thing with an eating disorder: you don't always know, and you can't ever assume, who may be struggling with food or addiction. If you've been through an eating disorder, perhaps you can spot it better than the average eye. There are certain key factors, behaviors and personalities that you are observant of from your own experience—the secretive ways of hiding to keep up your own struggle to control or suppress your emotions. However, the majority of the population will look at your weight and decide whether or not you struggle with food.

Remember, an eating disorder is an emotional struggle that affects the physical being—not the other way around.

So, for about a year, I struggled with bulimia once again, while living on my own in Miami teaching yoga full-time.

AUGUST 2015, MIAMI BEACH, FLORIDA

The official signing of our divorce papers were fairly straight forward, yet it seemed to take months to process in the court system. I returned my rings. I needed to purge and let go.

August is hurricane season in Miami, and officiating a divorce feel like a hurricane of its own. That same month, I was co-teaching an event called Transcend, in Coral Gables, just south of downtown Miami. There was a tropical storm coming through the same day of the event, which definitely didn't help our turnout. Among the three men who joined us, one I knew from a previous class I had taught. The other two, I had no clue. According to photos, one tall man with blue eyes wearing a bandana stood behind me in the group photo at the end. Although he never said a word to me at the event, he later contacted me on Facebook with a friend request and a follow-up message offering the use of his cameras, and to film any upcoming events I had free of charge.

Javier Olmedo. Friend request accepted.

Wow. Kind man. Nice offer. What did he want?

This Mexican character definitely did his research on me via social media and the internet. You can really find anything you want to find out about someone fairly easily these days, so its not like I was hiding too much. Like an open book (pun intended here), I've always been a believer that life is meant to be lived, learned, and then shared.

Javier had this concept and idea to create and produce a wellness travel show. He was a producer, pitching shows, and wanted to feature me as the talent and host. I love being on camera, and always have yearned to take the lead in a show, like the travel adventures I used to watch as a kid and young adult on the Travel Channel, Discovery, NatGeo, and via House Hunters International. I dreamed to be the next Samantha Brown, but less dorky and more depth, or like the late Anthony Bourdain, but a bit less dark.

Sara Quiriconi, Live Free Warrior, the traveling, storytelling, adventurous and health-oriented host sharing her experiences, learnings and reflections with viewers to inspire them to take that same journey!

I wanted to hear more, so we booked a time to meet over coffee and talk about this TV show idea he had.

JANUARY 2016, MIAMI BEACH

I was sick. Very sick. To the point I lost my voice and had a terribly stuffy noise and was wrapped in the layers of a down vest and scarf

116

to stay warm on a 70-degree weathered day. We met at a local coffee shop to look over the ideas Javier had in mind for this show. I was incredibly intrigued, and this man equally had my genuine interest as a friend. He was so easy to talk to, older than me, so I didn't feel threatened in the way that I did with other guys in Miami who knew I was recently divorced and back on the market, "available" for dating (terrible assumption, by the way).

Javier was different. When I was with him, I felt an ease to simply be me (head-cold and all), as we talked for what was scheduled to be a 30-minute conversation that quickly went past an hour talking about more than just the show.

I'm not sure how it was brought up, but he asked me if I wanted kids. My answer was, "I need to learn how to take care of a plant first before I even think about kids. But, no, I don't think so." I was honest. I was me; and it felt freeing.

I truthfully think I was sick and lost my voice from throwing up. It can happen, the scratchiness of your throat from the acids that rise from your stomach in the efforts to rid yourself of any food that is in there. Yes, I was still binging and purging at this point in my life. The 15-years I scoffed at in Marya Hornbacher's book? I surpassed that. Dealing with an eating disorder on and off for that many years, it proves that one needs to get to the truth and reason behind the disorder and the behaviors to understand and resolve it. The focus cannot solely be on one's weight or cessation of.

Javier and I planned the first date for filming our reel for the wellness show in March. It was a full day of filming with locations on Miami Beach and just south of downtown Miami in nearby Coconut Grove. A full day of filming that flew by in an instant, and I couldn't remember having that much fun or that many laughs in one day. I was given the opportunity to speak freely as I am and to be me, the silly kid, me the deep thinker, me the torn soul, me the sad blue eyes, me the jokester, me the movement junkie. It was me, just being me.

MARCH 2016, MIAMI

I was in between teaching yoga retreats; the first was in February, about a month back, in Turks and Caicos. The next one coming up was in May to Nicaragua, and was looking to be sold out by the time the travel date arrived.

I needed a break, I needed some Sara retreat time to pause and see what connection I could make with myself. I couldn't keep on living a life portraying wellness and self-care if I was throwing up to deal with my life. That wasn't living. Living a lie—that was dying, and another kind of cancer.

I had never been to Tulum, but the location interested me. There were so many yoga teachers leading retreats there, and I knew I wouldn't be hosting one there anytime soon. So, I might as well go check it out myself to add another stamp in the passport.

As a young kid, I went to the Riviera Maya of Mexico at least ten times. My grandparents had timeshares in Cancun, and we were lucky to be going every two or so years to vacation together as a family.

I knew that area of Mexico. However, I didn't know much about Tulum. I let Javier know in a text message that I had plans to travel there, and was going alone. Did he have any suggestions or recommendations?

"It's my country! Of course, I do!"

Intuitively, without thinking, and just from feeling, I said, *"Why don't you join me?"*

Javier looked up flights, times, and pricing, and sent them in a text message to me. I could feel his hesitation. My reply to him:

"RED BUTTON! RED BUTTON!," meaning DO IT!

Flight booked. Bags packed. La gringa y el Mexicano en Tulum, Mexico. ¡Vamos!

↗

CHAPTER 7:
LIFESTYLE, NOT A DIET

"The best and most beautiful things in the world cannot be seen or even touched. They must be felt with the heart."

– Helen Keller

This next part happens fast, and intensely. Even though this chapter only touches upon just over a year's length in time, the intensity of emotions, experiences, and changes that occurred were enough to motivate a new lifestyle for me—a lifestyle that would incorporate greater health, radical healing, self-discovery, self-awareness, and more passion that I had ever felt in my entire life prior.

Perhaps, then, maybe it's not time that creates experiences, knowledge, and self-awareness. Perhaps, it's more the quality of life and openness to feel, to being truthful enough with yourself to say, *"YES!"* and push your own red button. It is the choices and opportunities that arise in those key moments that can totally transform us.

MARCH 2016, TULUM, MEXICO

We were in a paradise. With a full schedule booked that Javier had organized, we swam with the turtles, explored a *cenote,* rode bikes through the grounds of an eco-resort, and a *temazcal* ceremony—at the *gringa's* request.

I had read about a *temazcal* in a recent spa and wellness publication. A *temazcal* is a traditional Mayan ceremony typically held in a heated clay hut shaped like an igloo. You have two tiny little doors: one where you get in and out of, and the other where they add the fire-hot stones. Some *temezcals* are just heat based. Others meanwhile, have a pool of water in the center. It's a Mayan sweat lodge wearing little to no clothing to purify, renew and spiritually cleanse yourself. Always one to try (almost) anything once, I was intrigued to see what it was all about, and I certainly could use a bit of cleansing to my spirit.

I arrived a day before Javier did. Prior to knowing he would be joining me, I had already booked a three-night stay at an Airbnb in the center of town in Tulum. The first night, I explored what was local, walking around town, grabbing groceries from the market and tasting the freshest guacamole I had had in my life from a tiny and quaint vegetarian restaurant, conveniently located around the corner from my Airbnb.

I sent Javier loads of photos of what I was up to, and texts throughout the day. Clearly, I was excited he would be joining. I had a friend, someone I intuitively trusted, and partner to share the adventure with.

In a last minute surprise, he had booked an available room at a beach-front property. This eco-resort was a 5-star luxury tree house, designed to disconnect from the world, and connect back with nature. A friend of a friend, who works in the hotel chain at the Riviera told him, *"You have to check this place out for filming your show!"* So, he got a room in exchange. And, Javier offered the room to me.

The night he arrived, we had the *temazcal* booked as well. I changed hotels and when I arrived, I was beyond blown away. Literally, the attention to detail and creativity of this hotel showed the work of an artisan. The wood is locally drawn from the native lands the hotel sits on, the structures are built around the tress to keep them fully intact and apart from the room environment, the view of the ocean from your own private balcony completely took my breath away—and, made me cry. I melt at the sight of a beautiful sunset.

Javier arrived late, after 9pm, and I was already tuckered out in the lobby asleep on a bench from a full day of outdoor exploration in paradise. To his surprise, he wasn't just filming the *temazcal*—he was a part of the experience too.

Together we had a private ceremony booked, and we were filming parts of it. That meant, we received the full treatment from the *Chaman* called in to lead the ceremony for us.

Three dreadfully hot hours later, I was baked, cooked, dehydrated and maybe cleansed? It was interesting to have an experience like this, but to do it with a man who was kind of a stranger, and in bathing suits? I later mentioned to Javier that I was slightly claustrophobic with a lung sensitivity to heat and humidity from cancer treatment. Things to tell your activity guide beforehand.

In any case, initially we had connected on Facebook, and now we were connected by a spiritual ceremony—what a start to this adventure together. Or, a premonition of what may come in our future?

I stayed at the resort, and he went to the Airbnb I had booked. The following day was a full outing of snorkeling with the turtles and *cenote* diving—two other things I loved doing in the past when I was younger. Play time!

We swam, filmed, laughed, and talked—a lot. This man could **talk**. Early on, I knew Javier had a lot of life experiences and stories to share. We talked about our histories, work experiences, life experiences, playful memories, future plans, and just about anything else in between. We felt incredibly comfortable together from the start.

The remaining two nights in the Riviera, we stayed in the same resort, about 30 minutes away north of Tulum, at an all-inclusive eco-reserve resort called *Hacienda Tres Rios,* meaning "three rivers" in Spanish. Upon check-in at the front desk, getting our bracelets for the inclusive access, I recall looking up at him talking to the desk attendant and thinking, *"I could get used to traveling with this man."*

That night, we caught the moon and the stars over the water. I started crying, while sharing a story about my grandfather with him. Who cries in front of a stranger?

Someone who isn't innately a stranger.

The rest of the trip was spent exploring and filming the Riviera together. We filmed on the beaches at *Hacienda Tres Rios* practicing yoga in a private little cove, took bikes out to explore the nursery and organic gardens of the hotel, and wrapped up the evening with a chefs' table dinner. Javier wasn't aware I had issues with food in the past, and the idea of eating 7 courses of different fishes freaked me the fuck out.

I was a good sport, and picked at or ate most of what was brought out in front of me. We still laugh to this day seeing the footage because you can clearly see I was uncomfortable eating some of the dishes. Ironically, food is something Javier absolutely loves, so he happily ate any of my leftovers. Balance.

It was an awkward night, and I had trouble sleeping. I felt a weird shift in my energy and was up through most of the night tossing and turning from thoughts in my head. What was going on? Why did this feel so weird, yet known? Was it completely inappropriate that I am here, in this hotel, on a trip with a man I barely know? And that we've shared so many intimate details about our lives with each other over the past two days in conversation? This entire experience—Tulum, the change-of-plans travel, new foods, trust and deep interaction with a "stranger"—was something I've never done before in the past. Yet, it felt incredibly organic, like it was destined. My inner emotions were conflicted and my mind unsettled.

The following day was my last, and Javier accompanied me to the airport in a taxi to wish me off while he stayed on in Cancun for a few more days, to meet up with a friend. In the car ride, I was tired from a bad night's sleep, and once we hit the main road back to Cancun airport, I thoughtlessly and with ease, lay down in his lap while he rubbed my back. Just like that, as if we'd done it a thousand times before in the past. I felt so very much at ease, and at home.

At the airport we had about an hour-long coffee at the Starbucks in the departures waiting area, sharing deeper conversations like I had never had in any relationship in the past. Who was this guy?

When it was time to head to my gate, he awkwardly kissed my forehead, and I took off through TSA security. I texted him before I got on the plane. When I was on the plane. When I landed. And, when I got back home, the words, "I miss you." I meant it in a friendly way, but maybe my heart knew something greater than my mind was ready to admit.

APRIL 2016, MIAMI BEACH, FLORIDA

Back in Miami, I was teaching and back to my usual schedule. And so was my eating disorder. I didn't hate my body the way I did in the past, but it still wasn't perfect. And, certainly, my life wasn't.

There's some irony, being a girl who suffers with body image and self-esteem issues almost her entire adult life, who then chooses Miami as home. Miami is one of the most beauty-centric cities in the world, known for it's grade-A plastic surgery and tanned, fit bodies—or, easier said, physical perfection.

I didn't move to Miami for the fake—I was in it for the palm trees, warmer weather, and *tranquilo* vibes. A much needed departure from the hustle and bustle New England demanded. For me, the ocean, the beaches and the feeling of the sun on my skin every day of the year felt like home.

I got a text from Javier (now called "Javi" at this point in our textual friend relationship) saying he had a rough cut from the video footage we filmed in Tulum and Playa. We planned to meet at a salad place in the middle of Miami Beach to review. Where we met, was neutral food ground. I knew their menu and would be able to order something.

After we ate, he pulled out his MacBook Pro laptop to show me what he had cut for a reel for our wellness and travel concept show. It combined footage from our first day of filming in March in Miami and the footage from our recent trip to Tulum.

I cried watching this video. It was me on film, and for the first time in a very long time I didn't critique the girl I saw in the clip. I wasn't thinking, ***"fat arms, look at the skin hanging over my pants, bad skin, fix your hair..."***

I cried because I looked at this girl and really liked her. I wanted to hang out with this girl, be her friend, and get to know her.

A combination of good filming and editing, yes, I'll give him that; but, it was also an "aha" moment for me to truly appreciate me for who I was. Javi was able to show me someone that I fell in love with: ME. He had captured ME on film, to show and share.

Tears gone, we quickly jumped from the profound and meaningful emotions behind the video, to silly jokes and being the silly little kids we were (are) at heart.

Finding my soulmate was the first step towards truly healing from my near life-long eating disorder and uncovering the person I am today.

Nobody believes, that up until this point, we didn't kiss or anything more than a friendly hug. We knew we were feelers, and emotionally intuitive; but, both us were fresh out of divorces and had our minds set on the idea that we weren't "ready" for a relationship, nor were we looking for one.

We were friends, but there was undeniable intrigue, and excitement. This was a person with whom I felt so instantly comfortable. The only other person with whom I had come close to feeling like this with was Len. But over time, I became acutely aware that I am heterosexual and wanted to be with a male partner, should the right man come along.

When I was ready, of course.

LATE APRIL 2016, DORAL, FLORIDA

You can say, *"When I'm ready"* but the universe and your heart may have other plans. When you allow yourself to feel it.

I had a private yoga client just south west of downtown Miami, and Javi offered me lunch at his apartment, just west of the city after. This beach and city-loving girl does not drive west of the city for anything aside from IKEA or the Department of Motor Vehicles—and for this Mexicano who offered to make me fresh guacamole, *"better than the one I had had in Tulum,"* he claimed—made me an offer I couldn't refuse.

The guacamole was good, but the kiss we shared after was better. We were on his futon in the living room talking as we had in the past, but the proximity between us, and physical pull was intense. When our lips first met, I knew in that moment I would fall in love with this man.

When something feels so right, and perfect, like it comes from another lifetime, you have to follow it. This doesn't happen for everyone, and I know this sounds like a typical love story. My intention to share this, however, is to allow yourself to *feel*. Forget numbing, forget the plan, forget what you should do, forget what you think you know, and you think you have to do—just *feel*. It will guide you in the right direction... to live free.

Here's where the timeline speeds up. Intense, yet real, and what felt right in every way. It was quality over quantity, warriors.

MAY 9 2016, TEPOTZLÁN, MEXICO

It was Javi's birthday, and he wanted to travel to his homeland of Mexico City and show me some of the outskirts. It was the first time I met his Mother, who kindly offered me coffee from the machine she had. I preferred Starbucks from around the corner, and my response was, *"No mames!"*—a phrase Javi had taught me, which does not translate very kindly when talking in polite conversation.

Ooops. We all laughed—Spanglish lessons for *la gringa*. It was perfect.

Driving out to Tepotzlán, we filmed at various locations and then stayed overnight at a hotel owned by a friend of Javi's in the mountainside. A celebrity spa and wellness resort, it sounded luxurious and beautiful. By fate, by luck, or by divine design, we had the entire hotel to ourselves. Really. No one else but one other woman who drank white wine the entire time was staying there. It was magical.

The morning of his birthday, we watched the sunrise in the empty dining area, cutting up our own papaya and fruit we had previously purchased. There really was no one in the hotel. It was perfect. We felt connected to everything around us, and it was exactly what we had chosen. That was the morning I fell in love with Javier (love number 4— the definitive love).

MAY 2016, SAN JUAN DEL SUR, NICARAGUA

I had a sold out retreat planned prior to our new relationship as a couple. I booked Javi to join me on the retreat. We went together, filming and sharing this experience now as boyfriend and girlfriend. Small room, tight quarters, mosquitos, howling monkeys, and a really incredible group of 17 yogis—one of which was my ex-boyfriend Pat, who was seeking some life-changing inspiration and decided to join.

Though it may seem incredibly strange that an ex-boyfriend would attend a retreat with me years later, I have been fortunate to keep a friendly and supportive relationship with a majority of my exes. I believe, when you connect with open, good-hearted people in your life—such as my relationship with Pat—and the relationship ends on a respectful note, it's possible you can still appreciate the past love you had for each other. Pat and I respected that we had served a purpose for support and learning for each other at an earlier point in our lives. Our relationship as a couple had ended when it needed to so we could both continue to thrive and move on. And to find our true soulmates.

Another example, Marco and I were able to do the same, leaving our relationship in a respectable manner, appreciating each other for the good times and life lessons we had shared. Having a puppy, and not children, I'm guessing helps ease this transition in our relationship. But it is a gift, to be able to have that post-relationship friendship with all of my exes. However, they're also friendships I've earned and chosen, with an intention to make happen by both parties.

I would imagine, as bizarre as it sounds, I could sit all of my three ex-loves in a room with Javier and they would all say the same things about my personality and oddball characteristics: childlike, intense, playful, loving, creative, exciting, and beautiful.

When you can genuinely be *you*, your truest self shines.

LATE JUNE 2016, MIAMI BEACH

Javi and I moved in together into a 2-bedroom, 1-bath spot on the beach. Not intentionally, solely by fate, we moved to an apartment right across the street from the area where we first filmed together in Miami Beach. When it's right, the circles of life guide you back home.

Javi and I were both signed into one-year leases with our previous apartments, but we somehow managed to sub-lease within a week to other parties.

All else going well, I still was struggling with bulimia. I had to make a decision, that if I was going to move in with Javier, that meant I had to move out with bulimia. My heart, and Javier, of course, won.

I'm not suggesting to anyone the best way to deal with an eating disorder is to move in with someone, or fall in love. It's important to note you need to fall in love with YOU first, then, maybe, the other half will follow. The objective was clear: I needed to heal me, and that was in the works. Then, I needed to work on the tactics, how I was managing. Moving in with Javi, was the final push I needed to finally let go of the eating disorder, and be me, and to live free from a cancer that had plagued me for more than half of my life.

At this point, Javier knew pretty much everything about my past. We honestly talked more with each about feelings, experiences, struggles and our souls together in the first few months than most talk about with their therapist over the course of a few years. We were incredibly open, and honest with each other about who were, where we came from, and where we wanted to be in the future.

In many ways, we were (are) complete opposites on the outside:

• Mexican/American

• Gen-X/Millennial

• Male/Female

• History of Obesity/History of Anorexia

• Spanish/English

• Kids/No Kids

• Pleaser/Warrior

However, we were (are) completely the same on the inside or interior:

- Emotional Beings

- Freedom-seeking souls

- Travelers

- Storytellers

- Creators

- Playful

- Passionate

- Wise for our years

- Ex-alcoholics

- Fitness-oriented

- Healthy eaters

- Dreamers

What if we, as a society, could feel deeper to find our connections, to focus less on the exterior? How much freer could we potentially be?

The truth is, we will all age and we will all change (more or less) over the course of our lifetimes. What we look like today will change tomorrow, and the next day, and the next year. We also all have the ability to learn new languages, fresh skills, and to adapt—if desired. However, if we're exclusively focused on external appearances and apparent differences, than we're missing out on the greatest guide and compass the human existence offers us—feeling.

Don't get me wrong, in a sexual relationship, I need to be attracted to the person I am with. However, that attraction goes beyond the physical exterior of what is perfection and what defines beauty. Attraction, and love, is a full-on manifestation of all of the senses coming alive, like a giant orgasm that doesn't need to be sexual, just sensual. But, we need to be able to feel first to find that connection. Luckily, I found my sense of *feeling.*

SUMMER AND EARLY FALL 2018, VARYING PARTS OF MEXICO AND THE U.S.

We traveled a lot together during this period for various work-related projects and productions, visiting Puerto Rico, Mexico City, Tulum, Cuernavaca, Las Vegas, Querétaro, Puebla, New York City, and in late October, Connecticut to visit my family.

In between, we talked about our future, what we wanted and how we would create that together. Javier and I knew ourselves best at that point, and knew that:

• We didn't want to have kids

• We wanted to live in the warm weather, opposed to the cold

• We felt more comfortable, at ease, and at-home with each other than ever before in our lives

• We wanted to share this life of "You can transform, evolve, and choose a healthier lifestyle" with others as a part of our purpose

• We wanted to travel the world filming, creating and sharing together

• And, we didn't want to do any of this with any other person in the world but each other

LATE FALL 2016, MIAMI BEACH

We had been together as a couple for only six months at this point.

After filming a kitchen clip together, featuring a "GUAC-OFF" (who could make *lo mejor*, or, the better, guacamole) *JUNTOSproductions LLC.*, our Spanglish Well-being and Travel content company, was born. The goal was to blend both of our worlds,—*Juntos*, to incorporate the Spanish word for together, and *productions*, the English component of our joint venture. Spanglish, *claro que si*, but of course!

We also decided to get married that upcoming January. Already having both been married, we wanted a small, intimate, and meaningful ceremony.

Javier and I decided *Hacienda Tres Rios*, on the river where we first traveled and filmed in Playa del Carmen, would be perfect for a very non-traditional *Chaman* ceremony on the beach.

↗

CHAPTER 8:
WHERE IS CANCER TODAY IN MY LIFE

"I wanted a perfect ending. Now I've learned, the hard way, that some poems don't rhyme, and some stories don't have a clear beginning, middle, and end. Life is about not knowing, having to change, taking the moment and making the best of it, without knowing what's going to happen next.

"Delicious Ambiguity."

– Gilda Radner

Cancer is like a tornado, that whips in to your life stirs you up, and spits you back out in to the big, giant world, learning how to rebuild, regrow, redevelop and trek onward. Cancer **changes** you—and that goes for any sort of major life transition or upheaval.

Where am I today, physically? I'm in the Riviera Maya of Quintana Roo, Mexico, writing the rest of the first and second parts of this book. I took this week off to focus, center, reflect, write, and breathe from the ordinary confines of the hamster wheel we put ourselves on when we're operating our daily routines at home. This, in itself, is something I never would have done in the past, to take a pause, a break, and say *"I deserve this, I need this time off!"*

This brings me to my next question: Where am I today, emotionally? Sometimes healing isn't just in a cocktail of chemotherapy. Sometimes healing is the swizzle stick of life. Can you to let go of control, trust in your intuition, speak when you need something, accepts what you cannot control, and have the strength to change what you can? Allow life to take control, to learn from the punches, to make the most of any hand that's dealt, to make the effort to be inspired by and interested in the most important person in your entire life—YOU!

By saying *YES*, that is the spirit of a live free warrior, to commit to thriving instead of surviving, and to choose to live a cancer-free life, because you're doing your best, as you desire, fulfilled in each moment. Because no one will choose for you the life you sincerely want to live. Every life lived is unique. No two stories are (nor should be) the same. This is your journey, this is your life, and this is your quest you're waking up to every morning. Only a true warrior—you, dear warrior—can do that journey and make that commitment for yourself.

JANUARY 2017, PLAYA DEL CARMEN, MEXICO

Javier and I were wed January 8th on the same private cove and beach that we visited on our first official filming trip together. Our wedding consisted of nine people in total. Most of us (myself included) didn't wear shoes. I had on a bathing suit under my simple, slip white dress. No veil, a beautiful tropical bouquet, and the simplest of matching wedding bands, handmade by a sustainably-sourced jewelry designer we had done a (ironic or not) wedding photo shoot with in the past.

There was no engagement ring, no bridal shower party, no engagement party, or bachelor fiesta. Our wedding ceremony was conducted by a *Mayan Chaman,* something my father asked for months after, *"Is this legal?"*

My incredibly supportive and open-minded family, I could only imagine the thoughts running through their minds when comparing the uniqueness of this wedding to my previous one to Marco. The experiences, and the joy shared that day, was far more important than anything tradition could have offered. To have my Grandfathers look down on us and open up the sky for a sliver of sunshine at just the right moment we were to begin the ceremony held outdoors on a day that was scheduled to rain all day. To keep the focus on the love we share, and our commitment to work at being better people for ourselves and especially together, in the light and honor of our families and the four directions and elements of the Earth was all we needed.

This is what mattered to me on that day. The rest, to me, was a show I already saw, and I didn't want to watch a repeat episode.

I knew what I wanted from the moment Javi and I initially connected. Whether my mind realized it or not at the time, my heart certainly did. Being open to feeling more and thinking less helped open me up to new ways of making decisions in my life. They became more intuitive, and less based purely on reason. Following my heart, following my feelings, and following my passions, the internal love, is what brought my soulmate to me. In turn, following my heart also brought me to my first and foremost soulmate: ME.

You can spend a lifetime searching for the ONE, but the one you need to find first in order to be happy with one else, is yourself.

JUNE 2018, PRESENT DAY

What has happened in between, and where am I in this present day, dealing with all of these previous "cancers" causing dis-ease in my life?

I'm still not perfect, and while some of the cancers have been eliminated from my mind and body, others remain stable, or in a non-malignant state. My job stress, physical health, issues with food, and marriage all still have their moments, not shining their brightest. With so many past emotions, and baggage (emotional, physical, mental), it's not so simple as to just surgically remove them. They are on a genetic and biological level by this point, more deeply, ingrained habits since childhood or even birth, still operating in my body, and my mind. The body can change, all for the better, but the mind does not forget. And, we mustn't forget, the mind moves the body.

Looking back over the years, my journals, and photos over the course of writing this book, it is evident that where I am today is a lifetime away from where I started.

The little girl who struggled to fit in, to be liked, to perfect her physical form, starved, drank, and numbed her feelings out—she no longer acts on those former crutches to pacify her emotions.

However, that little girl, no matter her age today, doesn't forget the lessons she's painfully learned. For it's these experiences that have shaped me into the person I am today, quite righteously.

What's different this time around is that I am more self-aware of who I am as an individual, who I want to be in the future, and I am committed to being a better person, seeking out opportunities, making choices, and taking action, to be the absolute best version of me for myself, my partner, and those I impact and connect with on a day to day basis.

In my marriage with Javi, I have found someone to whom I can commit to, yet also feel completely free. That came from years of hard work, radical self-honesty, and the courageous warrior spirit to be kind, yet firm, in what I wanted and didn't want in this life, including, but not limited to:

• I don't want to be throwing up every day of my life.

• I don't want to be waking up with a hangover each morning.

• I don't want to count every calorie that I consume.

• I don't want to weigh myself every morning, allowing the scale to determine my mood for the day.

• I don't want to work for a salary under someone else's payroll.

• I don't want to live in a town, or city, that I didn't feel "at-home" in (if even for the weather).

• I don't want to birth a child because I believe the world has plenty of other beings that need caring for; further, being a mother is something I simply don't desire.

And, I don't want to allow my body to be susceptible to another physical cancer or disease from the various "cancers" I had allowed to control my life in the past.

You can choose to be a victim of life, or you can choose to be

a warrior in life. In the same regards, the Big C can stand for cancer, or the Big C can stand for choice. What path do you for-C in your future?

(FUTURE) SEPTEMBER 29, 2018, 15-YEARS CANCER FREE

I haven't had my suggested annual set of exams—which include (but not limited to) a Breast MRI, Mammogram, Pulmonary Function Test, ECHO/EKG Exam, CBC, Thyroid level check, Physical Examination and Patient Assessment—since January 2014 prior to leaving Boston at Dana Farber Cancer Center where I had my last set exams and doctor check-in. I am probably due for a visit, and perhaps, after writing this book would be a good time to schedule it in.

Being naive doesn't fix anything, but neither does being afraid, fearful or anxious.

I'm not guaranteed to be cancer-free for life. In fact, I have a high risk of breast, or other cancers developing due to my previous Hodgkin's diagnosis, and the late side of effects of the chemotherapy and radiation treatment.

That cancer, I cannot control. I can only do my best each and every day to care for myself better than I have in the past.

What cancers I can control are the choices I make on a daily basis, with food, in my relationships, and how I choose to deal with stress and anxiety, and how I desire to live my life.

Death can happen long before a cancer diagnosis, when you're sitting on a hospital bed, waiting for an oncologist to give you your exam results. Death can happen when we stifle our needs, quiet our desires, think small, destroy ourselves, numb our brains, silence our minds, and ash our passions.

15 years ago, I was diagnosed with Stage 2A (possibly 3) Hodgkin's Lymphoma at the young age of 19. They never were able to tell me exactly what was the cause of my cancer. Deep down, I think I already knew. The real cause of my cancer was:

ME.

Taking full responsibility that it was a combination of all factors that could potentially go wrong to cause a mutation in a cell that would eventually take over the rest of my being.

Now, before this goes down a dark and dreary path, this is GREAT news! There is a huge amount of freedom and relief when taking responsibility for one's "cancers" in their life. If you feel you were a big part of the cause of your cancer, then you also know that you can be an even **bigger** part of the CURE for your cancer.

According to the American Cancer Society, approximately 5–10% of cancers are due to inherited genetic defects from a person's parents. This means that we are responsible and have freedom for a 90-95% chance of NOT developing cancer. With a healthy lifestyle, being active, removing toxins from our lives, decreasing stress, and eating well, we can create that healthier, higher percentage that can prevent disease from ever standing a chance of becoming a breeding cancer in our bodies.

So, take that power, learn all you can, invest in YOU because your well-being depends on it. You have the power, now you have the tools, and you always have the right, to the pursuit of health, happiness, freedom, and living cancer free.

"I hope this part of my life is one of the toughest areas I ever have to go through. But, if it's not, I'll just have to deal. I can live through life just trying to survive the bumps and potholes. However, I will be just "surviving life" not "living life" until I realize that the bumps and potholes actually are life." — September 2003

Perhaps cancer was the toughest part of my life. Maybe cancer isn't over for me. That's part of the risk that I'm willing to take. However, knowing the life I don't want to lead, just surviving, has led me to be clear and create the life I do want to live. It involves checking in with the following phrases that resonate deepest in my heart for the life I desire to create.

THE LIVE FREE MANIFESTO:

CHANGE WHAT YOU CANNOT ACCEPT, OR ACCEPT WHAT YOU CANNOT CHANGE.

I tried to change my body for years. In every single way you could imagine, just short of plastic surgery. In fact, the only "fake" thing on me, are my two front teeth after a trampoline accident as a stubborn pre-teen. I wanted smaller hips, to be taller, a tighter stomach, skinnier arms, perfectly straight posture, white teeth (that doesn't happen when you're bulimic for 10+ years), and the list goes on.

My hips? They're bones. They're not going to change. My height? Nope. Not growing anymore. Not at 34. My stomach? Well, I could do more crunches and abdominal work, or cardio, but that goes back to the "why" and intention of doing anything. My teeth are quite expensive, needing care and repair on a regular basis after years of destroying the enamel that protected them. The front teeth, however, are on the mend, getting implants for health reasons to remove an infection from an old root canal.

That's a short list of things I can, and cannot control when it comes to my physical being. Further, I can't control whether or not people love, like, or hate me. I can only do my best to be ME and to be around those that attract to the energy I naturally give off.

I cannot control whether a job I take will be a source of income for years to come, or if the position is short lived. What I can control is not being defined by a title, to diversify my skills and expand my network, and continue to follow positions that create and express to help my passions thrive.

I am committed in my marriage with Javier, and we've promised each other another 46 years together. However, there are absolutely no guarantees that we'll both be alive in 46 years; nor should we take our commitment for granted. A marriage takes work and effort, every single day.

I cannot control whether or not cancer comes back in a secondary form. I can control what I do on a day- to-day basis to be my healthiest, freest, and most stress-free (not easy for this Sagittarius) version of myself. And when I go off path, to not veer too far, but remember the end goal and stay close to be where I want to be—*that* is when I'm living free.

Mostly, it's losing attachment to labels, letting go of controlling a timeline that is out of my hands and simply doing the best I can to be a healthy me, making the best choices I can. A good marriage, a healthy body, and a life of living free are a string of empowered choices.

TAKE ACTION FROM HEART, NOT FROM EXPECTATION TO OUTCOME.

When I was in art school at college, I learned very quickly some creative projects will be successful, and many will be rejected. Not every piece will be deemed a success, yet art is also subjective to the eye.

In a way, relationships are like art projects, or paintings. Some will click and be a long-term investment, a painting you just *have* to buy, frame and display in your home. Others you can simply pass on, as they only catch your eye in passing.

Regardless of the outcome, a creative project, painting, relationship, or a homemade birthday cake, if your efforts came from good intention and from the heart, then you've done your best. It all goes back to the power of choice. We all have choices, at least two in every situation. What do we do with them? And, once we make them, how do we live with them?

I'm a believer and achiever of living without regrets. How does that happen? To be clear on what you want to learn from the punches that come along the way, and to take action on the opportunities when they arise. You can't move forward when hitting repeat on the same old track. Live. Learn. And make choices to help you move on.

IF YOU DON'T WANT TO BE TREATED LIKE A NUMBER, STOP OPERATING LIKE ONE.

For the longest time, numbers ruled my life. How many calories I was eating, how many calories I was burning, what grades I got, what my weight was, my designated hospital identification number, what my blood count was and if I could be administered chemo, how much my weight had dropped when I was going through treatment, and more. Later in life, during my 20's and the years living in Boston, it became about how much money I was making, what zip code I was living in, how much I weighed, how much I ate, and if I kept going on that path, it would have continued. Not anymore.

When I was a cancer patient, I despised being another number on the charts, to the doctors, and just another one in the cancer crowd. Technically, according to my clinical paperwork, I was "Unit # 120-13-98." I've become an apartment or a partial international phone number.

When I was laid-off, it was a harsh reality that I was a number to a company—another "unit" in the system that was no longer needed. It came down to a bottom line, budgets were being cut, and I was the next number on their list. It's what companies do. However, letting this rule your life is where the issues arise.

Today, I am secure that: I am not a weight. I am not a calorie count. I am not a salary. And, I am not basing my worth on what title I have at an agency or what the paycheck says at the end of every two weeks. In fact, I'm the co-founder of two LLC's, running a production company and personal brand, so there is no longer an agency and I happen to be the one writing my own paycheck these days.

If you don't want to be treated like a number, a "victim" of the system, then that effort starts with YOU, warrior. Value your self, care about your health over the scale, and tally smiles and successes—or failures, there are lessons in both—instead of calories.

COLLECT EXPERIENCES OVER THINGS.

Clutter, and extra things, always created anxiety for me. Nick-nacks, and items taking up counter-space, a massive overstuffed closet of clothing, or a desk filled with papers, pens and **THINGS!** I love to organize, to purge, to release and let go of what I don't need or what is in excess in my life. Disposing of papers, donating old clothing, having an empty, clear, organized workspace—this brings me peace, mentally, and creatively.

I'm very aware that this anxiety, a need to create order, along with the desire to purge, release and let go parallels the characteristics of anorexia and bulimia. However, this approach—to clean out unnecessary crap and organize—I believe, is a healthier mindset and method than I've had in the past. Minimalism and an appreciation for experiences over things is a lifestyle that is more emotionally, spiritually, and creatively fulfilling than any gift, shirt, diamond, or purchased thing could offer me.

How is this possible? It's the memories. And, when you're fully alive, experiencing moments, those moments don't leave you. The "things" are instant gratifiers, a temporary fix or solution to a deeper conflict or higher level of satisfaction. You get the newest smartphone, and you're super excited for the first day or maybe even week. What happens after? You have moved on, and maybe a reality about your finances, your relationship with your wife, or the dissatisfaction you have with your job quickly takes over that materialistic purchasing "high."

The involvements, the memories, and the feelings you feel during high-quality experiences, are the items worth investing in to create positive emotions that can physically change your chemical make-up. When you're on your deathbed (morbid, I know, but hang with me), will you really think back and remember that expensive pair of heels your purchased? Most likely not. But, you will recall that time you spent that new car money to travel to experience the Mayan Pyramids, and the one you saved your tip money to open the LLC of your own company.

Those are the experiences worth investing in. The material things, they'll just require more dusting on the shelves, or higher insurance.

DON'T SURVIVE. THRIVE.

Some facts: I was diagnosed with cancer just under 16 years ago. The moment you finish your last treatment, for chemotherapy or radiology, you go in to a stage called "remission." After five years of being free from the cancer disease, you are technically a cancer survivor.

The term "survivor" always seemed a bit dramatic to me. Read in the dictionary, to survive is, **"to get along or remain healthy, happy, and unaffected in spite of some occurrence"** (dictionary.com). To survive, to me, always sounded very victimized, like the cancer came after you in some awful way that was completely out of your control.

And it can! Truthfully, I felt attacked in many ways by Hodgkin's. However, the mentality that I was attacked also left me feeling less empowered. To be living and coping in the moment gave me more control over the actions I could positively take to counter the disease.

More importantly, after cancer, to say I remained *healthy and unaffected in spite of the occurrence*, as the dictionary states, is incredibly untrue in many ways. Had I remained unaffected, I wouldn't have chosen to eventually overcome my eating disorder, change jobs, remarry, and (eventually) write this book.

Cancer, as I mentioned in the opening of this book, doesn't just appear. There are causes, reasons, and genetics at play that create the recipe of its formation. Some are within our control, some outside of our control.

Cancer, like any challenge in our lives, has the opportunity to change us, to teach us something, and to help us become stronger from it. Like cancer, I decided that after any of these challenges, it was a scar, a battle-wound, and a reminder of the strength I had gained from the experience, and how I developed resistance. My life was no longer about surviving and just getting by; it was about becoming my absolute best, rising higher after each fall I took, and to continue living more fully, in each awakening day—thriving.

NEVER TRY. NEVER KNOW.

They said, *"Give yoga a try, you'll love it,"* during treatment. I said no way. 10 years later and I'm attending a yoga training to become a teacher—never try, never know. Had I said NO and never tried the practice, a few times, I wouldn't be where I am today, healed and recovered, from my addictions and cancerous habits.

Often times, it's fear that keeps us from trying something new. We pause or, worse, freeze in fear because what comes after is unknown. And, that *fear* scares us.

But, we can't let fear stop us from experiencing something that has the power and potential to transform us. Any opportunity or experience can teach us something, or transcend our being. We never walk away unscathed, if we're open, feeling, and living fully, being alive.

TIME IS ENERGY. ENERGY IS CURRENCY—AND TIME IS THE MOST VALUABLE THING YOU HAVE.

I read about the term *Energy vampires* a while back and fell in love with the concept. Energy vampires are people that we surround ourselves with, that instead of fueling us, they suck our energy away. We all have those people in our lives. After a conversation or interaction with one, we are left feeling empty, tired, and like we got hit by a truck.

Experiences and habits can do the same thing. Social media is a fantastic example of this, where we can go on just to check that one notification bubble that popped up on our phone. Next thing, we've lost half an hour in the endless scroll, where we've achieved nothing from, and we've been sucked (once again) in to the social media rabbit hole.

There are 24 hours in a day, or 1,440 minutes, or 86,400 seconds. At the end of that day you're not getting any of that back. No amount of money can turn back a clock (not even Botox), and the energy you're expending during those hours, minutes and seconds, cannot be returned back to you either.

Be wise in how you're spending it, as an investment in the output you wish to receive back in return. In reality, if I had the amount of time I spent counting calories, throwing up, hours working off a hangover, or moments concerned about whether or not some jerk was going to text me back, I'd have back an entire chunk of my teens and 20's back.

Busy isn't always a good thing, if being busy is simply filling your day with things that make the clock go tick. YOU have to tick, not the clock! You have to find those things that make you feel alive, and fill your calendar and agenda appropriately with items that give you energy, not take it from you.

PLAY MORE. THINK LESS.

Life can be so serious. When I was kid, I wanted nothing more than to be a grown-up, get a real job, and move out on my own to be like an adult. I'm sure I'm not alone in this pursuit, to be a kid and yearn for nothing more than to sit and be accepted at the "adult table."

Then we get older and we spend our paychecks chasing youth. Vacations equal freedom, Botox for youthful skin (not me, but so I hear), and caffeine for endless energy. What were we thinking as kids? I had it all backwards.

Yoga taught me to play a little bit more, and to take life a little bit less seriously. Honestly, is it really a big deal if you lose your balance and fall from a standing split? I didn't think so, and you're probably smiling just thinking and reading this. Yoga taught me life doesn't have space for perfection—that it can be messy, out of order, you can fall, find laughter, learn from it, and try again, a different approach—and life still moves on.

Cancer isn't anything to laugh about, but I do think it's important in any dark moment to remember the things that make you feel alive, laugh, and like a human BEING instead of a human DOING. While I was going through treatment, I loved going to the beach, surfing when I had the energy, learning in my classes at the university and going to the movies. It's important to find the *play* in every day to balance out all of the thinking we do on a daily basis.

Think of it (ha, gotcha there!), the only time our minds are not thinking are when we're sleeping. That's a lot of energy going towards the brain to figure things out! The mind operates on logic, while the heart moves from feeling and emotion. There's a reason we try to connect the two, like in yoga, for a mind/body connection. However, sometimes the heart and feeling needs to override any logic for passion, play and creativity to flow.

Part of the reason I love to travel so much is travel's ability to take me out of the routine and into the places that are extraordinary. That element of "play" to explore, get lost and discover keeps me inspired and out of my head—ahem, and away from anxiety and allows me to figure out everything in the moment as it happens.

Tapping in to my inner child, the one that yearns to be free, play outside for endless hours, laugh at stupid jokes, play tricks on others, and blow bubbles out of my nose—she makes an appearance more these days.

REPLACE THE WORDS "SHOULD" AND "HAVE-TO" WITH "OPPORTUNITY" AND "CHOICE."

You **should** have a kid. You **have to** make more money. You **should** work a Monday through Friday job. You **should** grow your hair long. You **have to** buy the luxury car to be successful. You **should** eat less and cut back. You **have to** lose weight to be skinnier or prettier.

Damn. Think of how many times we hear these words from others, say these phrases to people in conversation, or put them in our thoughts in our minds on a daily basis. A LOT, I'm guessing!

When we use the words "should" and "have-to" we're giving away all of our power. We are no longer making a decision but accepting what is proposed. It's a fuzzier version of reality that will leave us blind to the doors that are really open in front of us.

Now, replace the above phrases with the words "choose" and we have an entirely new mentality and approach.

"I choose to have a kid."

"I want the opportunity to make more money."

"I choose to grow my hair long."

Now we're sounding strong, empowered, and like we're the authors of our own books. Remember, warriors aren't puppets, and you're the author of your own life to live, because no one else has to live it but you! Shoulds will only get you to live someone else's ideal version of what life is. A life of shoulds certainly won't be living a life of your own.

JUST START, AND KEEP MOVING FORWARD.

There will never be a perfect moment to begin. The hardest part of graphic design for me has been that "Apple + N" to open a new document. Sometimes that blank page just stares at you waiting for inspiration to pop out of the curser like a magic trick.

Each choice is a blank page, and you hold the pen (or the mouse) that will create the first element.

All forms of yoga and movement that I've been drawn to in the past have emulated water. I'm dually certified as a 200Hr teacher, taking two similar, but different approaches to yoga sequence structure. The first training taught me anatomy and the basics for creating a flow. The second taught me how to be "fluid" and less defined. Later, Budokon taught me how to move the body and offered the inspiration to create my own transitions in an endless flow that allowed the creative expression to be free through grace, strength and movement.

Today, what I practice is a mix of everything that I've learned through trainings and my own mat exploration over the past 10 years. Starting a self-practice, yoga flow, or design project can feel like that. Where do I begin? What comes next? I'm lost without guidance, or a step-by-step. Trust yourself.

When we feel stuck, hesitant, in fear or doubtful, the biggest leap is just to start, to flow, and see where it goes—without looking back. We may fall, again, and again; count the rises, instead of the falls, to leap and create the net that will appear.

NEVER SETTLE.

Think back to the last time you filled one of those satisfaction surveys titled, *"How would you rate your experience?"* The bubbles, or online form, offer the suggestions: Excellent. Good. Satisfactory. Fair. Poor.

You select satisfactory. The experience wasn't mind-blowing, but it also wasn't a disaster. It was average. It was mediocre. It was what you expected. Nothing more. Nothing less. Good enough.

How many of your life decisions or actions fall in to this category? Good enough?

The jobs I left, the marriage I opted out of, the apartments I was living in, and even today, the jobs I'm selecting: many people's first question to me was, *"Why? Why leave? It's good, no?"*

Good enough. That doesn't cut it for me. If I feel stuck, stagnant, like I know I am capable of more or something or someone is a better fit for my own personal growth, to aim higher, or will take a bit of work to do something that's a better fit for me—I won't settle for anything less.

Life is way too short to make choices that are simply enough or satisfactory. Good shit takes time and effort, and that's where the warrior kicks in. I know this. My health took work, it took effort to quit drinking, it took effort to stop throwing up, and it took a hell of a lot of effort to move down the East Coast, divorce, be on my own, figure out who the hell Sara was, to then find myself to be where I am, with the man I'm with, and love, today.

EXCELLENT things take time and effort. Don't settle because life demands a bit of energy. That's why you're on this Earth! To grow, to learn, to move, to rise, and to make the effort to strive for excellence, because you deserve and will receive exactly what you settle for.

QUALITY OVER QUANTITY.

Something happened over the years in modern America where "more" started to equate to better. Bigger homes, more clothes, a larger wine collection, bigger bank accounts, larger diamond rings, and bigger muscles (or boobs).

I used to think a workout had to be over an hour long, and a yoga practice had to be 90 minutes in a studio. To be successful, I needed a paycheck over six-figures. Having all of those items on a checklist meant the quality of my life had to be great, because it had more and many of all the things that were supposed to add up to feeling good.

On a personal level, I wanted everyone to like me. Everyone. I didn't know how to deal with an acquaintance, a co-worker, or a family member not being particularly fond of me. Part of that caused me to mix, mold, and get lost in who the hell Sara really was, living by the expectations of the shoulds and have-to's that I mentioned earlier.

Today, I prefer to focus on the quality of an action, a relationship, a job, or any interaction or exchange in my life. I focus on how these interactions make me feel, and the quality of their energy, rather than how much I'm getting from it.

I don't need a big home, but I need a space to be creative, free, and safe. I despise having a "full" closet and prefer to have less, but better pieces that express who I am, who make me feel warm, and fit their purpose.

Yoga is a daily practice, however, the "practice" can be a stretch before a flight, 20 minutes in the gym, or a full on 90 minutes getting lost in a flow on my mat in my apartment.

The time I spend with my family is important, and even though we live in different states now, the quality of the time we share is better than when I lived in at home. Same goes for my marriage, I seek that quality time with my husband, where we talk about deep subjects such as learning from our past mistakes, falls, and struggles, to then laughing like two little minions about a prank one another played.

It's not about the calories, but rather the quality of the foods I'm consuming. Some will argue a calorie is a calorie; however, I can hardly believe that a day's worth of candy totaling 2000 calories is going to be processed as a day's worth of fruits and vegetables. Just a like a car, receiving the right octane of fuel is important for it to run properly, not necessarily that you're filling up the tank with $20. It goes beyond the numbers, and puts the focus on the quality of what's being consumed.

Lastly, I don't have a lot of friends in my life, and I don't need everyone to like me. The quality of a select few who really get me—ME—is what's more important. Not liking the Sara I pretended to be for so many years, but the real me, who is loud, direct, funny, smart, a kid, a business woman, and a bird who doesn't stay in one place for very long at any given time.

You don't need a lot. You just need a few, a few that are *awesome.* Dedicating your time, your energy and your SELF to those who are providing the maximum awesome—or QUALITY—will offer you the best return on investment you can entrust in.

IF YOU WANT TO CHANGE THE WORLD, YOU FIRST NEED TO START WITH CHANGING YOURSELF.

Being in the pediatrics section of the hospital and going through treatment hit me hard. It was way better than being in the adult oncology section (even though we did receive the occasional unwelcome clown party). However, seeing the babies and kids with no hair, sick in a bed, pale, thin, and visibly ill, and not playing or laughing was tragic.

I wanted to help. I was 19-years old at the time, and felt that even though I was one of the fellow cancer kids, at least I had a childhood.

It gave me perspective. Hopefully, many of those same children are now 19-year olds living a full life. At the time, I needed to focus on healing me, my self, from the cancer, but more-so from the other cancers in my life—the eating disorder, low self-esteem, lack of passion, and borderline (self-diagnosed) depression.

You can't fill up other people's cups if yours is empty. Start with building YOU to be the best you can offer others.

The second part of this phrase in the manifesto relates to our ability to judge others from the outside, when to let go of control, and other times when its best to just not give a fuck.

It's easier to tell someone else to "just eat" or "find a husband" and "you should..." These are all projections, and ways we can offer to "fix" the people and world around us. We can't do that job. It's not our work.

What is our work? Ourselves. Leading by example can be the best way to inspire others to change. But the desire to change has to come from within. NO ONE was stopping me from throwing up and forcing me to let go of my eating disorder. And, no one was going to tell me that maybe I was drinking a bit too much; perhaps, I should cut back?

That desire to change had to come from within, to want something better for myself, and to lead a life that is more purposeful and fulfilling. To inspire someone you care about to change, lead by example, share experiences and offer to be there when he/she may be ready to listen.

THE BEST BOOK IN THE WORLD IS A PASSPORT FULL OF STAMPS.

I was very fortunate as a child to travel every year, many times to another part of the country, and on the occasion, traveling to Mexico or parts of the Caribbean. I was blessed with these opportunities to see other cultures, how they operate, how different they were, and how I changed as a person from these memories and experiences.

Today, I am equally blessed, and making it a lifestyle, to travel the world, speak in other languages, meet people with unique backgrounds, hear their stories, interview them about their histories, and to add more stamps in my little blue book than I could have ever imagined.

You can read about a culture online, look at photos, and scour over history books. However, to really learn a culture, you need to walk the path, talk the language, taste the foods, explore what's seasonal, and respect the differences. That's transformational travel, and how seeing the world can change you on a deeper, soulful level.

Travel can open your eyes to see that we are all so different in our cultures and nationalities, yet very similar on a human BEING level. We all want to be happy, healthy, and LIVING FREE. Be OK to get out of your comfort zone, get lost, and reflect on what you find, and if it feels good, share that experience with others. It's far better than a book, or a postcard—share the experience of being.

159

YOU HAVE THE POWER TO CHOOSE ANY LIFE YOU DESIRE TO LIVE.

I wasn't a victim of cancer. I wasn't diseased by alcoholism. I wasn't a martyr of an eating disorder. And, I wasn't a sufferer of a divorce.

These were actions that were choices, side effects, or a result of a lack of information in my own life to cope and deal. Stepping out of being a victim to your own life, in to the warrior spirit, gives you the pen to write the next page.

I know these are hard words and honest opinions to share, but that's the kind of thinking that took me out of a dark place and started to offer me the tools to create the light to dig my self out. It's empowering to know that you are not helpless, alone, without choices, and lacking the knowledge on how to take that next step.

What is EMPOWERING is to believe that you can choose, you can create your own life, and you can be passionate in the life you desire to live.

Really. You do. Start believing it. When you're ready to start creating it, living CANCER free, head on over to the next part of this book for the workbook section to begin your own personal transformation. Ready to begin, warriors?

PART 3

THE WORKBOOK
LIVING {CANCER} FREE

↦

LIVING {CANCER} FREE:
WORKBOOK INTRODUCTION

"I am not here to give you a dogma—a dogma makes one certain. I am not here to give you any promise for the future—any promise makes one secure. I am here simply to make you alert and aware—that is, to be here now, with all the insecurity that life is, with all the uncertainty that life is, with all the danger that life is."

— Osho, *Courage: The Joy of Living Dangerously*

Part 3 is broken down in to four chapters. In each chapter I will share with you the tools that I used to transition from Part 1 to Part 2 I shared with you in this book. The chapter headlines will look similar to those used in Part 2; however, this time around, in Part 3, the work is up to YOU, warriors, to make the effort and make the changes to live free in your own life.

This workbook will offer you a "deck" of 52 tricks or tips to keep up your sleeve for those moments you need them the most to thrive beyond mere survival and rise above toxic cancers. Some of these tools you may use on a daily basis, some only occasionally, or on an as need basis. Like a deck of cards, these tools and exercises are there for you to keep in your back pocket, because when overcoming emotional cancers, it's always good to have an Ace up your sleeve.

Why 52? Because there are 52 cards in a playing deck, and I like to believe making strategic changes and taking leaps requires a bit of calculated courage and a touch of risk. This deck of tricks will help guide you there, and perhaps can be your own deck of tricks when you need one—or a full hand—to find that guidance or courage to play the table.

> *"...basically courage is risking the known for the unknown, the familiar for the unfamiliar, the comfortable for the uncomfortable, arduous pilgrimage to some unknown destination. One never knows whether one will be able to make it or not. It is gambling, but only the gamblers know what life is."* — *Osho, The Joy of Living Dangerously*

And, while we cannot always pick the hand of cards we've been dealt, we certainly can choose how we play them.

Another reason I chose 52 tips for this section of the book is there are 52 weeks in a year. It can be more approachable for some of these strategies to take one a week, making change gradually over the course of a year. Baby steps still move you forward, and success is a staircase, not an elevator.

First, in Chapter 9, we detox and clean out cluttered areas in our lives, and begin to research the things we are potentially passionate about. With a clean slate, we move on to Chapter 10, where we begin creating connection within ourselves, tapping in our intuition, while exploring some of the passions we've put on the back-burner. Chapter 11 is where we begin to incorporate things that nourish us. With a clearer sense of who we are after working through the previous two chapters, it is far more effective and efficient now to add in joys, healing tools, and actions that make us feel alive, and free.

The last chapter, Chapter 12, reviews the manifesto of Living Free and the ways you can apply it to your own life with self-inquiry and action. There is no one magic recipe that will heal all. The intention is that these tips and tools can be combined, traded or tested out to see which works best for you, and which one makes it worth that leap of faith that will take you to that place where you are living free.

Within this workbook, I'm not going to teach you how to beat your eating disorder, how to overcome your addiction to alcohol or drugs, how to move on from your dead marriage, or how to quit the job you hate and find a career of passion where you make tons of money.

The person that will teach you all of those things will be YOU, and perhaps, a team of professionals, if needed, to guide you to a place of health and wellbeing.

> *"It is not a sudden leap from sick to well. It is a slow, strange meander from sick to mostly well. The misconception that eating disorders are a medical disease in the traditional sense is not helpful here. There is no 'cure.' A pill will not fix it, though it may help. Ditto therapy, ditto food, ditto endless support from family and friends. You fix it yourself. It is the hardest thing that I have ever done, and I found myself stronger for doing it. Much stronger."*
>
> *— Marya Hornbacher, Wasted: A Memoir to Anorexia and Bulimia*

What this workbook will teach you is how to feel, how to be intuitive, and how to connect with your emotions. The food, the addictions, the wrong relationships and stressful jobs are tools or masks for the deeper emotions we're fearful of facing.

I'm not a doctor. I'm certainly not an oncologist. Nor am I a nutritionist, dietitian, shaman, spiritual healer, or a guru.

I'm a person, simply that, who's been through a lot of shit in her life, lived through them, learned a thing or two along the way, and now wants to share what I've learned with you. I don't have the answers what will work for you to keep you "Cancer Free" because there are way too many variables to factor in, and life doesn't come with guarantees.

If cancer taught me anything, it's that life does not come with any guarantees. So, we as a society need to stop looking for them. I know, there are no guarantees, that even my cancer, or any secondary cancer, won't make a comeback. That part is out of my control.

What I can control is what I eat, how I move, the thoughts I think and the choices I make on a day-to-day basis. Within my control is doing the best damn job I can to be cancer free from life, and enjoying as many "free" moments of it before I take my final savasana.

Lastly, here's a truth:

You will fuck up.

You may need to fold. There will be moments you want to drink, to throw up every last bit of food in your stomach, to starve out the emotions that hurt you or pain you deep from within. It is incredibly normal to have those moments and setbacks and desire to fall back on former vices.

Certainly, there have been those moments for me in my recovery. In very small cases, the old vices win. In the majority of those moments, the healthier, more empowered, and "live free" choices have won. Here's another truth: the more the live free choices win, the more they will gain momentum. And, like a pendulum, there is nothing that can stop it once its force has power and potential.

"Every object in a state of uniform motion tends to remain in that state of motion unless an external force is applied to it." — Newton's First Law of Motion

Newton was right. My last, and most recent, tattoo is of an arrow on my left forearm with the initials "l.f." scripted in the middle of it. An arrow, to gain momentum, needs to be pulled back in the bow in order for it to gain velocity and force. Once that potential velocity has been pulled back, it has the utmost potential to propel its way forward. In life, in recovery, and in risk-taking, sometimes you need that pull back in order to gain the greater momentum to propel yourself forward.

So, no matter the setback, no matter the fuck up, and regardless the vice, never lose sight of your target. Use the momentum you can gain in those moments of pulling back to propel you further and stronger towards where you CHOOSE to be moving forward in your own life, warrior.

CHAPTER 9:
DETOXING YOUR LIFE

Like any organized closet, it's important to take out what we no longer wear, need, or find that fits us, in order to make space for the new "wardrobe" that we're creating. In terms of life, we need to remove the cancers, the toxins and the energy vampires to make clean space to begin adding in new passions and purpose.

Let's get started with the DETOX tips first to clean out some of the space we'll need in the upcoming chapters for choice and change.

1. DETOX YOUR SOCIAL MEDIA

Still browsing your ex's profile on Facebook? Seeking out the competition on Instagram? Scrolling through endless photos of your former high school clique?

While all of this "comparing" and social stalking can be healthy to some degree, if it causes you pain, anger, or leaves you feeling like poo, it's time to clean out your feed.

UNFOLLOW or UNFRIEND as you find fit. If you need a plan, aim to clean out 5-10 a week, until you find your news-feed is nothing but positive people, memes and inspiration for the life you want to live. In essence, you start to create your virtual reality, because it's not really reality anyway—we know this. The beauty of social media is we can form and create our own reality and news feed. We have choices of who's posts we can see, and can equally choose who's post we don't want to see.

I call it the social media meditation process. In meditation, we learn to clear out the mental thoughts in our mind's feed that aren't serving our greater being (stay tuned for details on the mind in tip number 5). We can do the same thing in our social feed, cleansing and cleaning it out.

It's important to note, we can't run from reality and unfriend everyone just because they post something that isn't positive. That's not what I'm suggesting here. This tactic is for the energy vampires and draining follows that reap of us valuable energy and self-worth time and time again. We all know that "Negative Nancy" out there that will find anything to complain about in life. She's a good one to unfollow. The guy we continuously compare our less than amazing life to? Unfriend him too. Your energy is way to valuable to waste comparing yourself to someone else's *un*-reality.

2. DETOX YOUR INBOX

Think of how many emails you get in a day that you don't even read and just hit "delete"? There's another option for that chunk of emails: unsubscribe.

We sign up for a newsletter for some reason for a click-bait free download in the past, or we've been auto added from a form we filled out at the dentist office. They send emails a lot—like, every day. Instead of hitting delete, take the two extra sections to select unsubscribe.

Set a goal to unsubscribe to 5-10 email subscriptions each week until that number starts to dwindle.

Something I love about our digital society today is that at least deleting emails doesn't waste paper. However, it can waste your time. So, cut the spam and junk mail out, and let your inbox be a source of necessity and inspiration for messages that will fuel you, not deprive you.

3. DETOX YOUR ATTACHMENTS

Close your eyes and imagine a day without your cell phone. Not so bad, right? You'll probably maintain your sanity, and life will go on—in your head, at least. Now, reflect back on a day where you actually didn't have your cell phone or thought you lost it somewhere. Still that cool, calm, collected person you envisioned?

Nope. You were probably a hot mess frantically wondering where your life had disappeared to, spending hours to relocate it so you could reunite once again. Or, maybe I'm just talking about me here, and a past case where I lost my attachment to life.

Perhaps it's not a phone, but think for a moment: What are you attached to? Is it a material object? Is it a job title at work? What would you be without it? Detaching from your attachments starts with awareness, and then working through the conditioning around it.

Tip: start with one attachment, and refer back to the following process gradually.

Once you are aware of your attachment, grab a piece of paper and write down the answer to the following: What feeling or emotion does this attachment bring for you? What security does it give you? How does it boost your ego? Do you show it off to others with pride? Does having that attachment make you feel more attractive, wealthier, intelligent, or even spiritual by owning or wearing it?

Be honest with yourself in the above questions. There are no right or wrong answers, only your own truth. Once you're done with the questions, take the paper, crumple it into a little ball and toss it away. Close your eyes and imagine that item doesn't exist anymore. Notice any emotions that arise, or fears that start to build.

Then, ask yourself the following: does the safety of this item hold you back from taking leaps forward? Have you ever sacrificed any part of your relationship to it because of it? What freedom are you sacrificing to keep that item? Most importantly, do you want to continue this level of attachment to this item? If so, continue forward. If no, how can you minimize that level of attachment, or even remove it entirely?

Repeat this exercise over and over as you find beneficial, choosing different attachments, or even working through the same, if you need to. The idea is, to find freedom and cleansing by removing things we attach to. In the case of the phone, it brings me connection, order, memories, and safety. If I lost the phone, I could certainly get a new one. While I can't detach from it completely for the sake of my job and lifestyle, I can minimize how much I need to be on my phone and set boundaries and limits for social interactions, browsing and emails.

What is my job title today? Well, I lost the official title when I got laid-off a long time ago. Today I'm an entrepreneur, heading the titles of a CEO, CFO, Creative Director, VP of New Business, graphic designer, and (of course) author. These are self-proclaimed titles, yet highly earned ones. Each title, or hat, shifts based on the day's, or client's, needs. So, there is no attachment to any one in particular—the title presents itself based on the task at hand. In that case, doing my absolute best is my only 'attachment' these days, as a personal—and professional—moral obligation.

Is health still an attachment for me? This is an important one for me, one that I almost lost, and is one attachment worth fighting for.

What will you detach from in order to gain more personal freedom and to lighten the weight and load?

4. DETOX YOUR RELATIONSHIPS

They say we are most like the 5 people we surround ourselves with. Hopefully, those 5 people are very important to us and inspire us to be the best possible version of ourselves.

More than likely, they're not. Otherwise, you may not be reading this section of the book. Some people we can't nix out of our lives (immediate family members and our bosses can fall into this category), but we can limit our time with those who drain us and maximize our time with those that inspire, mentor, and support our beliefs, dreams, and mindset.

Think of 5 people you are currently surrounded by the most. Observe their characteristics, personality traits, mannerisms, current roles in life, and their future aspirations. Do they align with yours? Be honest here. Now, consider 5 people in your community or reach that do inspire, support and/or can mentor you to be better. Invite one of those people out for a coffee or lunch sometime, have a solid conversation about your goals and intentions. Make it a point to listen and learn from this person too; after all, there's something intriguing or inspirational about this person that you want to connect to. Observation is one of the best ways to learn and absorb the energy of someone else.

Side note: You will lose friends as a result of your changes. When you change your lifestyle or habits, you will challenge other people around you in a way that perhaps they're not ready to see. You will distance or lose these friends. However, think in the long-term. To surround yourself with the support of those who get it, who have similar mindsets and lifestyles, will allow you to move forward *way* further being encompassed with these kind of like-minded souls.

5. DETOX YOUR MIND

Call it meditation. Call it mental floss. Call it awareness. I won't get fixated on titles, because I've learned from the past, calling anything mediation can leave some people with pre-existing ideas of what meditation is and have them running for the hills thinking they're too real for this new-age kind of spirituality.

Listen up: meditation can be nothing more than focusing your mind on one thing at a time. Stare at your pen on the table, and that's meditation. Focus your mind only on the thought of the sand melting between your toes as you walk in the sand, and that's meditation. Hear only the sound of your own breath as you lie in bed first thing in the morning, and that's meditation.

Meditation doesn't have to be anything fancy, with a cushion, an alter and a Buddha staring at you while you're holding mala beads in one hand. That doesn't make you any better or more of a "yogi" or a better meditator just because you have the gear. What does make a good meditator is someone who practices. Not just for 10 minutes in the morning, but all day long. How does that happen?

Mental awareness.

It is said that we have 50,000-70,000 thoughts per day, this means between 35 and 48 thoughts per minute per person. That's 50,000-70,000 opportunities for that little light-bulb to go off in your brain.

Of course, many of these thoughts are subconscious and passing while others, not so much. Throughout the day, observe the thoughts that pass through your mind. Are they positive? Are they critical? Hear how you talk to yourself, what words you use to reference YOU in your own mind. Observe what you think when you look in the mirror, when you wake up on a Monday morning, after a workout and when you come home from a long day and receive a hug from your husband.

Observe all of these thoughts. Keep what serves and fuels you. See if you can detach or remove the negative ones that only pull you down. If there's a negative thought that pops into my head, I first question, "What facts support this thought?" Most of the time, negative thinking stems from emotion, not fact. By focusing on the factual information, we can weed out the emotionally driven BS and stick to what's real.

6. DETOX YOUR HOME

A home is a nest and a sanctuary—your peaceful space where you can let go, unwind, undress and just be you. Let that space reflect the cleanliness and pureness you want to be surrounded by.

Something happens with time, and we collect and stockpile *things.* One candle becomes seven, gifts from relatives of collectives they found while traveling add dust, and the Amazon Prime book addiction adds some unhealthy weight to your bookshelf. Cleanse, learn to let go, and weed out what you're not using or no longer need.

Here are a few ideas to get you started with detoxing your home. Don't try to accomplish all of these in the same day either. Start slow, tackle one room at a time, and create an organized plan to accomplish cleaning all of the necessary areas of your home over the course of a realistic timeline.

- **Kitchen:** Gadgets can be fun, but they also take up drawer space. Each time I move, I tend to let go of some old spoons, pans, or broken dishes. Instead of waiting to move at the end of your lease, do a kitchen sweep of gadgets and items you're not using and give them a second life to a friend who's getting in to cooking. Or, to a local soup kitchen or charity organization. A clear kitchen is one you'll want to cook in.

- **Bedroom:** I like an organized space, free of extra knick-knacks and things cluttering up white furniture space. Baskets and drawers can be a big help for hiding some items you need (extra blankets, for example) but don't necessarily always want to see. Have some pillows, but don't let them fill your zen space. Keep a few items that hold memories or bring you peace near your head or on sideboards. For example, I have a Ganesh, a pumice stone turtle from Greece, a few black and white photos I took in Aruba and Santorini, and a small side lamp for reading at night. Keep it simple, but intentional, leaving your dreams space to expand. Last, set a weekly schedule to clean your sheets, bedding and towels so it feels fresh and welcoming

- **Closet:** As a general clothing rule, if you haven't worn it in a year, you probably won't wear it. For household items, instead of piling things up in your basement, dispose of things you're not using before giving them a second home. Sometimes I feel bad giving away things, or selling them to a third party via online apps; however, I ask myself, would someone get better use out of this than I am? There are a lot of people in the world who could use this. If so, I let it go.

- **Bathroom:** I'm just as guilty of buying new products and leaving half a jar of cream in the back of the cabinet. For my other fellow product junkies, take a regular, inventory of what you have, what you can toss or donate, and what you need to keep in the front to use up before buying something else. Beauty products have a shelf life too.

- **Office:** Remove clutter and keep it organized. We'll go into greater detail on office space in tip number 11 coming up. For now, if you work from home or just have a space sectioned off to drop the mail and pay bills, keep that space clean and organized. This way, nothing gets missed and it doesn't become an eyesore, keeping it a zone for productivity and for getting things done.

- **Refrigerator/Cabinets:** Does it smell? Toss it. Is it in a paper or plastic container from leftovers? Let it go. Are the peaches rotten at the bottom? In the trash. Go for simple in this category. Keeping the refrigerator stocked with fresh vegetables and fruits is a dream, but not always easy for everyone to do. Have on hand some greens, some easy to prepare cruciferous vegetables (broccoli, cauliflower, brussel sprouts) and in-season fruits that you can eat with your hands for a snack. Fresh produce is always best, but if you have to, you can get flash frozen as a last resort. For frozen foods, if it has ice caked on it, it's freezer burnt—toss it. Cabinets, I keep a simple stock of some grains, a few canned (no salt, all organic) beans, plain salsa with no additives, raw nuts (keep these refrigerated), and a mix of ground grains or oats for random recipe inspiration. There's no cereals, fake foods, white-processed anything in my cabinets. I honestly could go on for an entire chapter on this section, but I'll offer you a condensed version in tip number 8 a few pages ahead.

- **Living Space:** In general, I'm a huge fan of reorganizing a room with the items I already have, instead of feeling like I need to buy something else in order to refresh my home. It's like a creative puzzle I need to figure out, and it leaves me feeling accomplished and inspired, at the same time. Before you need to buy that new end table, take everything out of the living zone. Grab a piece of paper and map out two or three different layouts of how to make the existing furniture, plants, and items work. Get creative with what you already own.

7. DETOX YOUR MEDIA CONSUMPTION

Under the "media" category, I'm specifically referring to both social media and TV consumption. There are mixed studies out there that will suggest social media can actually qualify as an addiction; however, I'll say at least, social media can develop into a very time-consuming bad habit. Ditto that for TV.

Often, we'll go on autopilot when we're watching either. The scroll of a smartphone is the same "click, click, click" of a television. We browse, in search of something to entertain us, or numb our minds, to transport us from our current reality and living life.

Instead of numbing your mind, empower it. One of the best things we've done in our household is actually not have a TV. In the age of OTTs (Hulu, Netflix, Amazon, YouTube RED), the need for a TV is diminishing. This can be great, but online media can also be worse. Binge watching shows, spending hours up late at night finishing just the next episode to see what happens. That's no better than the "click, click, click" of a decade ago.

Limit your time spent on both social media and watching TV/OTTs. One hour at night, being selective in what you're browsing. If, after 10 minutes of searching you don't find something, grab a book and indulge yourself in some reading instead. We all know this will help you sleep better than staring at a screen anyway. Maybe it's a book (this one included) that will educate or inspire you on your new passion or that career you want to leap towards. That spark of inspiration won't happen when your mind is numb watching mindless media.

8. DETOX YOUR KITCHEN

Hate me or love me for this one, we're about to get real about how to detox junk food from your kitchen. Remember the goal you set when cleaning this area, that you're dedicated to your health, not your taste buds and habits. Ready to begin?

Toss:

• Sugars, brown honey, syrups, fructose, dextrose

• White bleached flours, white bread, white rice, white pasta, muffins, pasta, bagels, rice cakes (white rice based ones)

• White potatoes, flavored oatmeal, and most packaged cereals (which contain added sugars or bleached, processed grains)

• Jams, jellies, sugar-added peanut butter (most of them have it added), jarred or canned fruit in syrup or with added sugar

• Sweetened drinks, commercial juices, sodas

• Alcohol (it converts to sugar, FYI), or limit to only meal times (to avoid a sense of total deprivation here)

That's a very short list of things to rid your home of to fuel and feed yourself the best you possibly can. It's not possible for everyone, I'm aware. Start small, with one category each week and gradually detox your food if that helps wean you into changing your taste buds.

I'll delve further in to foods to add in to your healthy lifestyle in Chapter 11, where I discuss nourishing the body. Instead of focusing on what you're leaving behind, look at all the healthy options you'll be adding in—not to mention, the added years of life and health you'll be adding too!

If you want to take the above list a step further, I also remove dairy and animal products (particularly meat) as well. A vegetarian or vegan lifestyle isn't for everyone and I'm not here to convince you to give up your *moo*. However, I will note, if you do a quick Google search with the search terms, "study vegan diet cancer" you will see the results weigh heavily in favor of a vegan diet to prevent cancer and reoccurrences.

9. DETOX YOUR BODY

Commit to move your body once every day doing something that FEELS good. This exercise isn't for the calorie burn. Find an activity you like to do that leaves you feeling energized after, not ready to indulge in an extra serving of dessert because you've "earned it."

What you've earned is the ability to continue to move your body, to stretch it, flex it, care for it, and keep it healthy. I read a quote recently that said, "Exercise is a celebration for what your body can do. Not for punishing it." And, if you're in it for the long-term, creating a healthy relationship and mindset around activity and exercise is crucial to sticking to it.

Here are a few ideas to get you started with ways to move every day:

- Take a walk outside during your lunch break.

- Practice 10 minutes of yoga in the morning to wake up.

- Unwind at night by stretching in your bed for 15 minutes to get a better night's rest.

- Attend a yoga class 2-3 times a week.

- Commit to working out 45 minutes before your work day. Or, after.

- Try a new class each week to keep it fresh and challenging your body in new ways.

- If you're traveling, make it a point to check out the gym or fitness center in the hotel first thing. Moving your body is the best thing you can do after flying or being seated for an extended period. There's no reason to lose your healthy lifestyle just because of work and travel. With so many options we have today for fitness in your room, on your phone, hotel gyms, classes, and day passes, there's absolutely no excuse in this category in my book—and in my life.

10. DETOX YOUR EXCUSES

One of my favorite personal sayings is:

Learn your excuses and get smarter than them.

Excuses. We all have them. Some are small, keeping us safe in our bubble of complacency or being kind to not hurt others. Others are big, and a lie we tell ourselves, preventing us from moving forward to change our sails to cruise on forward.

Notice the difference between the following scenarios.

"Ah, I really can't make it Friday night to your party, I already had other plans!" Which is a much kinder way of getting out of going to a party that you have no interest in attending, and a fairly harmless excuse.

The other, more often excuse we tell ourselves is: "I'm really just drinking to calm my mind down a bit" after finishing off your 5th glass of vodka. It's no longer "calming"—I've been there. It's binge drinking and it's the kind of lies many addicts, and those stuck in fear from changing a habit, tell ourselves to make our choices and actions "OK" in our own minds.

It's rationalization as we are lying to ourselves.

One of the best tools I've worked with in the past is writing down a list of my excuses that I tell myself:

• "I'll start eating healthier tomorrow."

• "If I'm alone tonight, I know it's an opportunity to binge and purge."

• "It's Friday! So what if I go out and party? Everyone else is!" I've also said the same thing on a Thursday, Saturday, and Sunday too.

It's a small list, but these are some of the excuses I used to tell myself in the past to mentally assure myself that my habits were OK and completely normal when in fact they were bizarre and unhealthy circumstances.

The worst part is, believing these lies I told myself only harmed me more. I wasn't able to move forward to make healthier, more empowered decisions until I became aware that the only person I was really hurting and lying to was myself.

Knowing your excuses, you can then make plans to be smarter than them. Meaning, if you know you're more likely to put off eating healthier tomorrow just because you overate during lunch, instead of waiting until tomorrow to start a better habit, write down exactly what you're going to make for dinner to create a healthy meal for you. Or, another option, make plans to meet a friend at a healthy restaurant, someone who is into a healthy lifestyle and jointly committed to eating well that evening.

If you know you are more likely to binge and purge on a night you're alone, plan to do something special for yourself that evening. Take YOU out on a date for dinner, a movie, book a pedicure, or indulge in a book at a coffee shop, or while people watching.

Learning where your faults are isn't a bad thing—it's a GREAT thing! It is incredibly empowering to know the moments where you're most vulnerable to make an "oops" because it's in those moments that you can begin to make a choice to learn and live free instead.

11. DETOX YOUR WORKSPACE

Whether you work from home or you work in an office, keeping a clean, clear and orderly desk space allows for creativity and inspiration to flourish. No matter how much desk space you own, having less clutter can keep you focused and even more energized.

As a general rule, cleanliness = productivity.

Here's a few tips to organize your workspace:

• Keep only what you use on a daily basis on your desk.

• Organize office supplies in drawers, and then drawer organizers.

- Use a filing system for papers or project folders you need in sight (bonus for going eco and digital and not using any paper).

- Remove any distractions from plain sight.

- Make your workspace a food-free zone. This not only keeps your keyboard clean, but it also allows you the space to pay more attention to how much and why you're eating, instead of mindless eating.

- Dedicate 10 minutes on a Friday afternoon to clear up and to give your desk a cleaning prior to the weekend. When you come back to it on Monday morning, you'll feel a bit more inspired and ready to kick off the week with a fresh start.

- Have a trash can nearby to dispose of any waste papers, instead of letting them pile up.

- Scan it, and then recycle it, including papers, documents, temporary photos, etc.

- Minimize incoming clutter. Do you really need that magazine or catalog? Or, is it necessary to print out that large document you need to sign (yep, there are digital apps and programs for that)?

- Think vertical, and place a spacer underneath your laptop or monitor to create a small cubby or drawer underneath it for additional storage.

- Ensure you have the proper lighting for working effectively. Natural light from a window is best, but that's a tough one to expect in most offices. You can buy a lamp for your desk and use an imitation light that mimics the rays of the sun.

- Add some greenery. A small plant on top can be a delightful touch, and creates positive energy.

12. DETOX YOUR HARD DRIVE + OLD MEMORIES

In today's digital era, it's incredibly easy to snap photos, save, and upload. There's a saying in my family, *"It's digital—we can delete it!"* So we tend to take way more photos, many of which, I never end up using for anything.

Now, being a producer, I have way more video files than photos, which are larger, heavier, and take up far more space than any old .jpg would. I make it a point to cleanse and clear out my computer, hard drives, and smartphone of old photos, videos, or messages that are taking up space, holding bad memories, or keeping me stuck in the past that will take me nowhere in the future.

The same goes for social media memories. If you have a lot of photos of you and an ex that keep popping up on your screen as reminders, maybe give that box a little *"hide and show me less reminders like this"* and set some of your old albums to private, or even delete them if you find it liberating in some way.

I am not suggesting delete any bad memory in your life or laptop just because it doesn't make the highlight reel. Quite the contrary, I have many old photos of me from college days and after graduation very intoxicated and emaciated. These are certainly not my fondest years, nor most memorable; however, keeping them serve a greater purpose for both the documentary I'm creating, and as reminders of how far I've come in my life. In a way, they're inspirational for me.

Letting go of old photos, bad memories, or files that don't serve your healthier lifestyle and warrior path can be liberating and freeing. That "letting go" and deleting action can feel like the deepest exhale as you hit "Empty Trash" and say goodbye. A purging, a release, a weight that you no longer need, cleaning out your hard drive of bad memories leaves space for the better ones that you're creating for the future.

CHAPTER 10:
DEVELOPING CONNECTION

This area of the book takes a lot of effort because it requires change. We're replacing old habits with new ones, and that is never an easy task. Change and transcendence demands mental and physical effort. Not only are we focused on altering our actions, on a deeper level we're also switching up our thought-process and ingrained ways of thinking, many of which, we've been doing on auto-pilot for years. The brakes we need to apply here need a little force, and a heavy dose of getting clear on our WHY.

So, that's where we'll begin. Getting clear on your WHY.

13. CONNECT TO YOUR WHY

Your *why* is like a seed of a tree. Each branch, each limb and each leaf stems from and connects back to that seed that grew into something greater. Questioning and getting clear on your why, or a reason for wanting something, from the beginning offers a navigational tool towards change. There will be many moments where the sails of your hopes and dreams will get pushed by different winds. Navigate with your inner compass, warriors, towards the direction you're aiming for and no winds can steer you off course.

One of the hardest moments for me when overcoming my eating disorder, especially bulimia, was that trigger moment of, "I can keep eating, zone out my mind, and then throw it all up if I want. No one's home, I can eat and easily get 'rid of' whatever I consume. In that moment, and with any trigger moment for any addict, or anyone looking to make a change, is when *we always have two choices.* We can:

1. Act from habit, and we already know what will happen, or

2. Act from our intention, or our WHY.

If I know my *why* to be healthier, and to no longer act on bulimia as a tool for turning my mind off, using food as a numbing device, I can make a choice based on: valuing my health, deserving to feel nourished, the desire to wake up with a fresh mind, shame- and guilt-free, and be energized from a restful night's sleep.

Having all of this clear in my head, I (over time), became more likely to pause, connect with my WHY first, then ask, *"Are the following actions in line with my WHY?"*

This took time, many failed attempts, but gradually the why and the will became greater than the habit.

Today, write down your why for wanting to change some aspect for the better in your life. Get as clear and specific as you possibly can, including details, people, feelings, emotions, times, locations, and any other specifics that will help you be as clear as possible for the moments you have the choice to make an empowered decision, rather than acting from habit.

14. CONNECT TO YOUR BREATHING

Breath is your simplest, most basic need over anything else to live. Even before food and water, you need to be able to breathe to be alive. It's also one of the first things we forget, and the last thing we focus our attention on throughout most of our day.

Why? Well, we, as humans, are incredibly concerned about the past ("should I have said or done this instead?") and our future ("what ifs...?"), more than the present and our breath. In turn, our mind isn't able to connect to either of those places, our past or our future. Our breath, when we're focusing on it, is solely in the present moment.

The incredible power of the breath is something that we can all benefit from. Breath goes well beyond the focus and benefits of meditation.

Try out the following three breathing exercises (also called **Pranayama**, if you've heard it referenced in a yoga class) to aide in stress release, better focus, and deeper rest. All of these exercises you can do for a mere 60 seconds to experience even the slightest benefit. However, 3-5 minutes in total would be the recommended amount of time to commit.

1. INHALE/HOLD/EXHALE/HOLD

This one is best for stress release, and I employ this breath with my eyes closed and connect to visuals in my mind. Find a comfortable position in which you can breathe easily in, take a full inhale and exhale naturally. To begin, inhale as slowly and deeply as you can. When you cannot inhale any more air, hold your breath. While holding your breathe, it's important to not tense your body, but to soften what you can (including your face, shoulders, hips, and mental images of whatever stress or knot you're experiencing in life at the moment). Begin to visualize what is holding you back or standing in your way in the moment of breath retention.

To finish, slowly and with control, exhale all of your air. On the exhale, imagine yourself moving past that limitation, beyond and achieving the next step towards your "success" (the same one you were visualizing in the first exercise). When you cannot exhale any more air, hold your breath on empty. Notice whatever thoughts or emotions come up when you're holding your breath. Observe your mind. Inhale when ready, and repeat this cycle, 4-10 times.

In arguments, traffic, CT Scans, or triggering moments, I find this breathing exercise to be the most beneficial. All of the aforementioned are moments of stress, and by focusing the mind and the breath on that stress to do the work to release it (the "cancer" emotions) and let it go, I'm less likely to hold on to that stress within the body.

2. CLEARING SPACE

Gently close your eyes, shift awareness from the external world to your physical space and breath. After a few rounds of organic breathing, begin extending the length of your inhales counting to six, and your exhales to six.

Repeat for 8 rounds or so, and then release your counting. With a clearer mind, begin to focus on your end "success" goal. Visualize what it would feel like achieving that goal, what you would be doing now in that moment once you are there, and what thoughts you are telling yourself, having achieved that result. Begin to embody the exact person in that position you are seeking to be.

Continue this extended breath and visualization for 5-10 minutes.

3. IN 4, HOLD 7, OUT 8

The magical sleeping tool, this one helps to calm my mind, especially in those 2am wake-up-out-of-nowhere calls. Dr. Andrew Weil is famous for this one, but one I use whenever I'm tossing and turning for too long and need some quality sleep.

From any comfortable seated position, inhale to a slow, complete count of 4. Hold the breath to an even count of 7. Exhale with control to the count of 8. Repeat four cycles of this breathing, repeating another cycle if needed.

While I didn't learn or practice yoga or breathing exercises when I was going through treatment therapy, I would imagine this would have helped me immensely in moments of receiving chemotherapy, on the radiation table, and in the CT and PET scanners where you're enforced to sit completely still and "relaxed" for extended periods of time. These days, I use this exercise not just in bed, but also when I'm at the dentist or other similar "stress-induced" environments where I am required to sit still or in uncomfortable situations.

There are numerous other breathing exercises, too many to list in this short segment of the book. However, start with these general, accessible three and enjoy the benefits of breathing and breath awareness. Then start your own exploration and path of learning other techniques for an extended toolkit of breathwork for any situation where we need to just breathe.

15. CONNECT TO YOUR OWN SONG

Think of a few words to describe your life, your personality, and your outlook on life. Personality traits are simply actions, attitudes and behaviors to describe us, as individuals, and we, as humans.

If you struggle to find these words on your own, ask trusted and respected friends and family members who know you and treat you well and who can be honest to help get you started. Another idea, I've posted the question **"What are three words to describe me"** on Facebook and was overwhelmed by the incredible response others had to share with how they saw me. Having a few select words that best highlight YOU can help you remember your true strengths in times where you may feel your weakest.

Once you have these words collected, choose 3-5 of them that best resonate with you. Make it a song, create a personal mantra, or stick them on a post-it that's tacked to your bathroom mirror to see every morning when you wake up. Let the words be your song of fight, of strength, and of self-love to keep pushing you up in lower times.

Here's a short (long) list of positive personality traits to get you started:

Active	Creative	Gracious	Organized	Serious
Adaptable	Cultured	Hardworking	Original	Sexy
Admirable	Curious	Healthy	Passionate	Simple
Adventurous	Daring	Helpful	Patient	Skillful
Agreeable	Decisive	Heroic	Peaceful	Sophisticated
Alert	Dedicated	Honest	Perceptive	Spontaneous
Appreciative	Deep	Honorable	Perfectionist	Stable
Articulate	Disciplined	Humble	Personable	Strong
Athletic	Dramatic	Humorous	Persuasive	Studious
Attractive	Dynamic	Imaginative	Playful	Subtle
Balanced	Earnest	Impressive	Popular	Sweet
Brilliant	Educated	Independent	Practical	Sympathetic
Calm	Efficient	Innovative	Precise	Tasteful
Capable	Empathetic	Insightful	Protective	Thorough

Captivating	Energetic	Intelligent	Punctual	Tidy
Caring	Enthusiastic	Intuitive	Rational	Tolerant
Charismatic	Exciting	Kind	Relaxed	Tractable
Charming	Extraordinary	Logical	Reliable	Tough
Cheerful	Fair	Lovable	Resourceful	Trusting
Clean	Faithful	Loyal	Respectful	Understanding
Clever	Firm	Mature	Responsible	Uninhibited
Colorful	Flexible	Meticulous	Responsive	Unpredictable
Compassionate	Focused	Moderate	Romantic	Vivacious
Confident	Forgiving	Modest	Sage	Warm
Conscientious	Freethinking	Neat	Sane	Well-rounded
Considerate	Friendly	Objective	Secure	Well-read
Contemplative	Generous	Observant	Selfless	Whimsical
Cooperative	Gentle	Open	Self-reliant	Wise
Courageous	Genuine	Optimistic	Self-sufficient	Witty
Courteous	Good-natured	Orderly	Sensitive	Youthful

Browse through this list, collect your words and create your own song to sing (literally, or metaphorically) for the moments you need a boost and reminder of how great you really are.

16. CONNECT TO YOUR BODY

Mind and body connection is a phrase that is tossed around a lot in the wellness and yoga world, and can sometimes feel a little overused and watered-down from its potential. However, for lack of a more accurate phrase, mind/body connection can be a huge step in resolving negative emotions towards ourselves, and helping to unleash the power to heal years of self-esteem issues, eating disorders, and even addictions.

In my case, yoga helped to reconnect the feeling of my body, its strength and purpose, and to discover the desire to care for it once again. Learning to move and be strong, and recognize that my body wasn't just a "thing" but a verb, that was, and is, something that continuously evolves and changes on a daily basis.

Beyond yoga and movement, in general, here are a few additional exercises you can work on right in this moment to develop a calmer connection between your mind and your body:

1. Body Scan Exercise

You can do this one standing or lying down, but it is recommended to close your eyes as you're doing so. First, take a few rounds of deep breathing, in and out. Your eyes are closed, remember, so all of the "focusing" we're talking about in this exercise is actually your mind's eye doing the visual work.

Move in sequential order through the following list of points of your body. Pause in each one for 1-3 full breathes to relax and release any tension you may notice in that particular area. Perhaps you feel something, or maybe you feel absolutely nothing. Just keep breathing, without judgment or expectation.

The following exercise I find particularly helpful when going through any MRI, PET or CAT Scans, to relax your mind and body, remain focused, and help reduce anxiety.

When you're ready to begin, start focusing on the:

• Crown of head

• Cheekbones

• Jaw

• Shoulders

• Hands

• Upper back

• Lower back

• Hips

• Thighs

• Calves

• Ankles

• Toes

When you've gone through this entire list, you can either:

1. Go back up the body in reverse order.

2. Return to your natural in and out breathing.

2. Mirror, Mirror on The Wall

Standing in front of a mirror, look at yourself rather quickly and notice where your critical eye immediately takes you. Note your thoughts. What negativity does your mind tell you?

Then, close your eyes and for the next 30 seconds, continue to see that area on your body. Instead of the immediate negative thoughts that unconsciously come in to your mind, rewrite the script and tell your mind positive things about that area instead.

Recreate the story in your head by creating new neural patterns and ways of thinking by repeating this process over and over again. Over the course of a few days, weeks, or maybe months, you can begin to learn to trust the mirror and what your eye and mind see—together.

3. Hand Mantras

Seated or standing, begin by touching the tip of your thumb to the tip of your index finger. With each word of the following four-word phrase, transition your thumb to touch the tip of your index, then middle, then ring, then pinky finger.

Repeat the following phrase:

*Peace. Begins. With. **Me.***

If that phrase resonates with you, continue using it. Or, move on to:

*Peace. Begins. With. **Change.***

Again, if that phrase resonates with you, continue using it. Or, move on to:

*Peace. Begins. With. **Love.***

Last, but not least, when you're ready move on to:

*Peace. Begins. With. **Freedom.***

Work through one, or all, of the above phrases, repeating the one that resonates best with you 5-10 times moving through your hands. In stressful moments, I've found this exercise to help calm my mind, my heartbeat, and center my thoughts instead of letting them run off on an anxious tangent.

17. CONNECT TO YOUR CREATIVE ENERGY

"Art is never finished, only abandoned." — Leonardo da Vinci

When did we stop painting with our hands and drawing on walls with crayons? Fair enough, maybe not drawing on walls in our adulthood is saving us a ton of money in painting and interior design work. However, it's invigorating to tap in to our artistic side as teens or adults.

If drawing or painting isn't your thing, you're in luck. There are hundreds of ways to creatively express yourself, including:

• Fashion

• Music

• Movement

• Graphic Design

• Photography

• Writing

• Cooking

• YouTube Videos

To my fellow perfectionists out there, you don't need to be good at one of the above to actually do it. You just need to remove all judgement, make the time, and do it. That's the key to being creative: just do it, and see what you create. Maybe your painting turns out brown, or your cupcakes fall flat. Who cares! It becomes more about enjoying the process of exploring and trying out something new.

I call this tip *creativity experimentation* in action. Here are a few tips to help you get your creative juices flowing:

1. *Make a dedicated space* to create from.

2. *Keep it clean* and clear of clutter, papers, and anything not related to your creative project.

3. *Collect, or fill, your space with inspiration.* This could be mantras, colors, quotes, or a Pinterest board.

4. *Just do it!* It's easier to get stuck contemplating where the perfect place to begin is. There isn't one. Just now. And now. And, now! Those are the perfect places to begin: NOW!

5. *If you start to feel stuck, switch up your space.* Take a walk outside, take a yoga class, head to the beach, meet a friend for coffee, or check out a gallery. When you head back to your space, you may find that next creative kick to complete the project.

6. *Pick up where you left off.* After experiencing #5 and changing the energy space, review your project or piece from your first attempt. Maybe you still love it, maybe now you want to change or edit something. That's the process! Create, edit, change, create, and eventually save out, or export, your masterpiece.

18. CONNECT TO YOUR SUPPORT CIRCLE

There's a big difference between alone time, and feeling lonely in a negative manner. For the moments you're feeling down and lonely, like *nobody wants to play with you* kind of lonely, reach out and connect with your support circle.

Take 15-30 minutes going through your email/Whatsapp/text/facebook message list and write your friends, or even acquaintances, a quick note just to say *"hello!"* Typically, we tend to reach out to people only when we need something. Sometimes it's nice to receive a message to say hi and you were thought of—and it feels good to give those messages too.

To take this a step further, tell someone about your struggle or what you're trying to achieve. Make sure it's someone you trust, who won't judge if you fall or fail, but understands the importance of supporting you in your efforts no matter what. Let them hold you accountable for your progress, like a check-in, or be able to call him/her when you just need to talk through some feelings.

Creating and developing this type of support has helped me in the darkest trigger moments when I would want to act on my eating disorder or start drinking. Having people around you who know what you're struggling with and want to achieve—and want to see you succeed to overcome it—can be a game-changer for anyone looking to overcome addictions or issues.

19. CONNECT TO YOUR LIFE STORY

Sometime, a long time ago, someone told me that I should write a book about my life. Of course, I laughed at the idea at the time. But, here I am today doing exactly that.

Writing this book has helped me make peace with a lot of my past, histories, and memories. More than anything, writing this book has helped me heal and remember how far along this journey of ups and downs in life I've successfully made it through, and how much I've learned along the way. Writing this book has given me strength to continue pursuing unknown paths and has given me courage to keep pushing forward in the moments of doubt and to put in to perspective what really matters the most.

Even though I don't remember who encouraged me first to write a book about my life, let me suggest this: write the story of your life. Determine your "cancer" tipping point, defining your B.C. (before cancer) and A.D. (after cancer's death). It may be a phrase someone said to you, or a quote you read somewhere. Perhaps it's something larger, like a death in the family, an illness, or a transformative travel that shaped your thinking and perspective on life.

Write all of these moments, the highlights, and the low points in a story about YOU. Continue to update this story, because our life story is never really finished—only a work in progress. The benefit of having all of these notes will be in reading about these "cancerous" moments, or hard times, to better help you realize how far you've come and how strong you really are.

20. CONNECT TO YOUR SELF-ESTEEM

We all have moments where we're feeling down, low, or not so great about ourselves. That's life, and that's normal. However, staying there isn't a place we want to pitch a tent in. So, it's important to have resources from which we can pull ourselves up from that darker space and see the light once again.

Keep a folder file of things that make you laugh or uplift you on a down day. I have one of these on my desktop folder and it's literally called *"Things that make me smile."* I know I'll have those days that I don't feel super strong and I will need that reminder, *"Hey, stop being so hard on yourself, Sara! P.S. You're awesome!"*

Yes, the real work starts from the inside, not the outside. However, sometimes it's helpful—or even necessary—to have an objective perspective provided by a trusted friend or partner, rather than our own inner critic.

Another tactic to try on: when you're really feeling like poo, do the best to take care of you. I have a personal motto on days I feel down, and am sure to add in some ab work in my fitness routine, do my make-up to feel the most glam, and allow myself to eat all the fruit I want for the day (including dinner). These are all things I've realized make me feel better about myself, help pick me up, and are fairly harmless to me.

Start making a list of things that make you feel better that are neutral territory and keep that list handy on the days you need that pick-me-up.

21. CONNECT TO MUSIC

Music is a language, emotion and art all on its own. It can evoke nostalgia (Bon Jovi), happiness (Pop songs), tears (Piano or Instrumental), sexuality (Madonna), and even start a revolution (The Beatles). That being said, music is emotion, and can help us to tap in to a feeling that we sometimes cannot express in words.

Since I started teaching yoga many years ago, I always took pride and pleasure in creating playlists to accompany the classes I used to teach. The music that started a class had to be upbeat and inspiring, a slower pace towards the end of a flow, and for the end of class, savasana, a super mellow, low key number without words—all sequenced as such to create an emotion for the yogis.

Determine different moods, or emotions, that you want to tap into at certain times and create a list of songs that counter, or balance, that emotion. For example, you're feeling unworthy because a boyfriend just called it off with you. Or, in my case, I lost my job from a layoff and have feelings of not being good enough. Keep your esteem and self-love vibes high by creating a playlist of songs entitled *"You Are a Badass"* and list a group of songs that make you feel strong, like a warrior, and inspired to rise and keep pressing forward.

Another way to spin this tool: if you have a hard time expressing emotions (like I did for many years in the past, thinking I was a baby for crying), when you are in a stuck moment, put on some slow, sad, mellow tunes. If the tears fall, let them flow. Sometimes it helps to give yourself access to and allowance to feel and process emotion in a physical way; especially when we can't always find the words for them ourselves.

Most importantly, allow yourself to get lost in the music and FEEL. Bonus points if the music makes you dance—getting your body moving is a fantastic tool for releasing emotion and energy. More on that later.

Music inspiration can be found at @livefreewarrior on Spotify https://open.spotify.com/user/livefreewarrior

22. CONNECT TO YOUR INNER CHILD

Somewhere along the way in the aging process it seemed like a great idea to stop being a kid and start being more grown-up, or "adulting" as we call it today. Until you actually become an adult and realize, *"What the hell was I thinking?"* and we (as adults) work our asses off to have a week or two of vacation, and sometimes a weekend of free time to do whatever the heck we want like kids again.

Life Monday through Friday can involve a bit of that child-like play too. We just need to get a bit more creative and open our minds to make space, time, and effort to be that kid again. But, how can you be a kid in an adult corporate world? To answer that question, it starts with reflection.

I like to call this process the *"Benjamin Buttoning"* effect. Take a moment to reflect back to when you were a child. What were some of the activities you used to love doing. Maybe you loved playing baseball outside or dodge ball with a team. Or, you used to spend hours playing dress-up.

Find ways to add those "child" activities back into your life as an adult— and make the time for them now.

Perhaps there isn't a dodge ball game you can join, but there are adult sport teams or leagues you can sign up and get involved in. Or, make a weekly effort to head to the batting cages. If you loved playing dress-up, find an acting class in your area. Or, grab your iPhone or camera and make a weekly YouTube video to upload and share about any story you wish to act on and create.

The idea is, put in the effort to be creative. See how your childhood playtime can turn into adult playtime too. This will not only make you a more joyful, energetic person, but possibly more youthful and creative at the same time.

23. CONNECT TO YOUR VALUES

I've outlined in Chapter 8 how I founded and developed the *Live Free Manifesto*. This manifesto (also described in the upcoming Chapter 12, and posted in the index) is based on a set of my values and life's purpose.

Ask yourself, what matters most to you in your life? One day, when you die (hopefully not today, but it will happen someday) what will you reflect back on and care about or remember the most? I promise you, no one ever said they wish they had more clothes, lost more weight, or worked more hours at the office. Be honest, and get clear, with what things in your life you live for, that excite you, that fill your heart, and that make your soul dance.

Now is the fun part: write your own manifesto! Use small phrases as reminders of these values and goals. Here are a few examples to get you started:

"Travel the world"

"Family & Friends, instead over-time"

"Memories, more than shopping carts"

"Enjoy your meal, over counting calories"

Your own manifesto, or check-list, can help you in decisive moments whether something you're pondering or pending is inline with your list of values and beliefs, helping you determine if that choice is a *"Hell, yeah!"* or an *"I'll pass."*

For me, I know traveling the world, creating, sharing and taking part in experiences that make me feel alive—this is what matters to me in my life and what I want to achieve during my time here on Earth. So, all of the actions I pursue and take, I am sure that they are in line with those values, and help support the goals that I wish to fulfill in my life. Hence, the birth and evolution of the **Live Free Manifesto** and its role in my life today.

24. CONNECT TO YOUR EMOTIONS

Fine. Ok. Meh.

Being honest, none of the words listed above are emotions. Yet, somehow those words are what we use to describe how we feel on a daily basis.

To begin understanding our habits, and create newer, healthier, cancer-free ones, we have to take a deeper look at our emotions. If we can tap in to our emotions and begin to better understand what we're feeling, (and, even greater, what we're seeking) we can adjust the habit to get the same reward using different, "healthier" habits.

An emotion is defined as *"a state of feeling"* (Merriam-Webster's Dictionary). That being said, an emotion or feeling is not necessarily true or based on fact, but rather your own intuition and conscious understanding. In other words, emotions aren't necessarily real, and they definitely are not permanent.

The beauty of this realization is that if our emotions aren't permanent, meaning that they can be changed. Eureka! By being able to change the negative emotions, we can decipher what's real, what we want to keep, what we want to let go of, and what we want to change.

Start by building your emotional vocabulary. Learn how to connect to the power to change our emotion when we need to identify what's going on in the inside so as to heal, restore, and recalibrate our mental stream of consciousness.

The following is a budding list of basic emotions to tag on to:

SAD	ANGRY	SCARED
unhappy	mad	frightened
sorrowful	annoyed	nervous
depressed	irritated	panicky
miserable	furious	intimidated
down	enraged	alarmed
gloomy	cross	afraid
heartbroken	frustrated	fearful
devastated	vexed	startled
hurt	choleric	terrified

INSECURE	SUSPICIOS	HAPPY
unconfident	wary	cheerful
self-conscious	distrustful	merry
unsure	cynical	joyful
doubtful	disbelieving	pleased
hesitant	skeptical	delighted
timid	chary	gleeful
shy	mistrustful	carefree
introverted	disbelieving	buoyant
unsafe	dubious	untroubled

JEALOUS	HOPEFUL	LOVE
covetous	optimistic	fondness
envious	confident	attachment
desirous	positive	tenderness
insecure	sanguine	warmth
protective	cheerful	intimacy
vigilant	upbeat	affection
anxious	lighthearted	passion

mistrustful	buoyant	desire
resentful	expectant	lust

Here's an example:

Emotion: I feel lonely at night when I'm by myself.

Reward: I want to feel busy, occupied, or distract myself.

Habit: I act on my eating disorder, binging and purging.

Not a healthy habit, I'm sharing from personal experience.

Here's a healthier example:

Emotion: I feel lonely at night when I'm by myself.

Reward: I want to feel busy, occupied or connected to someone else.

Habit: I call a friend at 9pm just to say HI, or write in my journal about 5 things I'm thankful for today.

Get it? Now it's your turn. Next time you're in that cycle, feeling stuck in your emotions, figure out what you're feeling, how you want to feel, and what you can positively do to achieve that reward.

25. CONNECT TO SILENCE

Noise can be incredibly distracting and cause a lot of anxiety. Pair that with the "ding" "bzzzzz" or "Bzzt Bzzzt! Bzzt Bzzzt!" as your phone notifies you of the latest post, like, message or email and you've got an attack of distractions and unnecessary alerts to take away your focus and drain you of positive energy.

What happens when your computer crashes, or your phone starts to malfunction? You unplug it, turn it off, and give it a restart. Your mind needs that shut off point too. Be your own iDevice and turn off YOU every once in a while as well.

I suck at this one. Honestly, I do. But, that doesn't stop me from doing it (#noexcuses). I know taking breaks in my day is something I need to schedule in, in order to feel my best and not burnt out or overwhelmed. I make sure to schedule time in the morning for meditation, create space in the afternoon between calls, emails, filming and/or editing to read a book, go outside, or watch a show for 15-30 minutes. Food has always been tricky for me, so I do my best effort to eat in a calm, relaxed and spacious environment with good company, or by myself.

Yes, it takes effort, planning and self-awareness to make all of this happen. However, it's so worth it because you will feel good and balanced rather than on the go-go-go and burnt out, tired, and angry from overdoing your efforts.

Many studies have actually proven when problem-solving or creative thinking it's actually beneficial to shift your focus to something completely different to access that *"aha"* idea or brainstorm more effectively.

So, take a pause in the day, make it a point to indulge in a 15 minute afternoon siesta, and schedule in some iMatter time. Shut down, and restart.

CHAPTER 11:
CREATING A #LIFESTYLENOTADIET

"Food is not the enemy—food is energy."

— Sara Quiriconi, Live Free Warrior

Diets are like dating: you can go in to it knowing it will be a one-night stand; or you can be on the hunt for a long-term keeper. Chances are, when it comes to food, you're looking for something you can marry.

I could share with you in this chapter all the tips and tricks to lose weight that I learned and employed when going through an eating disorder. That isn't going to help you, instead, it would shackle you up to control you for the rest of your dieting life.

Instead, I want to focus on offering tips that took me out of that eating disorder and need for control and share ways to GAIN freedom through eating well for a lifetime of longevity, interest, and health.

26. NOURISH GRADUALLY

Changing your diet and your approach to food occurs gradually. It's not something that happens overnight, and while you can go cold turkey and clean out your kitchen vowing to only eat organic salads for lunch and dinner for the rest of your life, that approach typically doesn't create a life-long lasting change.

Instead, allow your body and mind time to open up to something new. Try one new healthier food habit a week. As you try it on for size, reflect on how your body reacts or changes, then adjust if you need to, moving forward with the next gradual healthier swap.

This takes time, energy, and effort, yes. But, I would be lying to you if I said one diet or pill could fix all of us. That's just not true. What works for my body isn't necessarily what's going to work best for you for a variety of reasons and variables. Therefore, for each of us, it's a process of trial and error to discover our own unique recipe and blend for true, healthy eating.

I've found it helpful to keep track of changes and results in a journal, scheduling in what I'm changing or trying, how I feel at the start of the week, middle of the week and end. Experiment, and make it gradual and fun, trying out new foods, categories, and dietary lifestyles.

Here's a sample of a journal entry to get your started:

CHANGE: _____   DATE: _____

NOTES BEFORE: _____

_____

_____

NOTES DURING: _____

_____

_____

NOTES AFTER: _____

_____

_____

KEEP THIS CHANGE: YES / NO   NEXT GOAL: _____

In my own experimentation process, I've discovered the most profound changes have been eliminating dairy and meat, and adding in more fresh fruits and greens throughout the day getting the majority of my nutrients from plants. About 90-95% of the foods I eat these days come without a bar-code or packaging. I'm not suggesting you go vegan, or plant-based. However, I am encouraging you to explore and observe what changes and adjustments you make that leave you feeling your best.

In the end, the "diet" or lifestyle title you choose doesn't matter— it's how you *feel,* and that it's a sustainable change you can make a lifestyle habit from it. Choose what works best for you. The fall-backs will happen, and in those moments it's important to write down your WHY—why you're choosing this healthier path and refer back to it every time you fall off track.

Last but not least, the best time to start a #lifestylenotadiet is NOW— not Monday, not tomorrow morning, not after dessert. NOW! Because LIFE—which is a part of your life*style*—is happening in the NOW, not the past, nor the present.

27. NOURISH THROUGH CRITICISM

I remember when I stopped drinking. One of the first things I lost, aside from my buzz, were the friends I had around me. Change challenges others. When you change, it makes those in your circle question their own actions and beliefs. If they're ready to change as well, then that's great news! You have a buddy to take action with and rise together. However, most need to discover that light and take that leap on their own time.

When you change your food, it's important above all to put yourself and your health first. People will criticize you—some will ask questions out of pure curiosity, while others will come from a place of judgment and defense. If these are people you can cut out of your life, refer back to Chapter 9 on detoxing your relationships and focus on surrounding yourself with those who will support and encourage you.

However, if these are people, like family, or co-workers, that you cannot just say, buy-bye to, here's a tip to help you in those challenging moments of confrontation or questioning.

Hear what they have to say. Really, open your ears, nod your head, and even repeat to understand what that person is sharing. Then, let it go. This is your food journey, and no one will be as self-invested in the food you eat than YOU. In the end, it's your body that is receiving the food, and in turn, the positive or negative effects. Consider this: a friend is drinking shots and eating steak and pasta for a night out on the town. He looks like he's having a great time and enjoying himself; however, what he doesn't share is the awful feeling of waking up with a hangover the next day and constipation from consuming the processed carbs or meat that get stuck in his colon. Gross details. Maybe true. Either way, the after effects are not healthy, nor sustainable.

Similarly, no one is as interested in what you purchase for your stock investment portfolio, the same goes for the nutritional "investments" you put into your digestive system. Invest in your BEST, and fuck the rest.

28. NOURISH IN THE "GRAY ZONE"

There's a tendency to categorize food in to good and bad foods, black and white thinking—this is the origin for many eating disorders, including my own. Categorizing foods in to good and bad and putting something off limits can set you up for guilt, shame and deprivation.

When I was anorexic, there was a large category of foods that were bad, or blacklisted. Anything with fat, high in calories or high in carbohydrates was off limits. What did this create? Deprivation, and in turn, it set me up for a binge and purge later in the evening when I would gorge on all the "no-no" foods, thinking I could just rid myself of them.

If you struggle with eating issues, perhaps you have experienced a similar deprivation and/or black and white mindset. Instead, I encourage you to view food as one big gray zone, where nothing is black or white, good or bad. Instead, view the gray zone as an energy detector, and each food has an energy rating based on how "alive" it is.

For example, an apple that has just been picked in the peak of fall in New England falls incredibly high on the energy level. In the opposite spectrum, a box of processed cereal tossed with sugar (looking not alive at all) would fall very low on the scale. I could go on with examples, but I think you get the point.

When food is alive, it has energy. That energy is what you're fueling yourself with. Similar to the people, relationships, jobs, and environments you choose to place yourself in, food is another category that can change your energies and aura.

Shift your thinking from food as good or bad and become a food energy detector, filling your tank with the highest octane out there when possible.

29. NOURISH BY CLEANING YOUR PLATE

Take a look at the average meal you're consuming for breakfast, then lunch, and then dinner. What percentage of the food that you're eating is "real" food? And, do you know what real food is?

According to research published in the *American Journal of Clinical Nutrition*, 61% of the food Americans buy is highly processed.* That is the majority of your diet. Yikes, that's a lot of fake food we're consuming! Within the study, highly processed is defined as, *"multi-ingredient industrial mixtures that are no longer recognizable as their original plant or animal source."* So, we're consuming food that doesn't even look like it's original form anymore?

To help change these percentages and get back to basics, begin the process of what I like to call *"cleaning your plate."* First, educate yourself on what fake foods are, learn about how foods are processed, and read up on where they come from. Do your research and learn about the fuel and creation of your life force—food!

Here's a short list of the top processed foods recommended to eliminate from your diet to begin the *"cleaning your plate"* process:

* *https://academic.oup.com/ajcn/article/101/6/1251/4626878*

- Granola bars (high in processed sugars)

- Frozen meals (loaded with preservatives)

- Canned soups (incredibly high in sodium)

- Ketchup (read up on the sugar count)

- Processed meats (who knows what's really in that loaf meat counter)

- White bread (processed and refined grains with little to no nutritional value)

- Sugary drinks (including sodas, juices, energy drinks, and sports beverages)

- Ice Cream (loaded with sugar—opt for a homemade banana blend in the blender instead)

- Chips or French Fries (baked, fried, it's all the same and no longer even qualifies as a potato)

- Margarine (engineered only to look like butter—it's not even real)

- Sweetened Coffee Drinks (You're drinking your calories here, warriors. Be honest—did you really think a venti caramel macchiato has any health benefits to it? Stick to black, unsweetened, or with a dash of non-dairy milk for flavoring if needed)

- "Low-fat" anything (removing fats from foods that typically have them occurring naturally in them—for example, peanut butter—simply removes what could be healthy fats and replaces it with added sugars, which naturally has no fat)

Read labels, do your research, and clear out your plate from foods that only come with bar-codes; the fewer the ingredients, the better.

30. NOURISH WITH SIMPLICITY

Dove-tailing off of tip number 29, eat more foods that have less packaging. The best kinds of foods are still in their purest form—the ones that come without a bar-code. Why? Because they don't need any packaging covered with advertising and marketing slogans to sell you on them. A ripe, shiny, sweet smelling orange doesn't need a fancy ad to make you buy one. It's perfect and naturally desirable as it is.

That's not to say all packaged foods or those with a bar-code are bad either. Many fruits and vegetables come with a sticker and number for purchasing (self check-out anyone?). Instead, I would recommend you place an emphasis on learning the psychology of the supermarket setup and educating yourself on how marketers target and advertise to YOU, the consumer.

Recall your last trip to the supermarket. Do you remember the sweet smell of the bakery or rotisserie chicken? Did you pass by fresh cut flowers cornered next to the neatly displayed produce section as you first entered? How about, did you **oops!** get more than you originally went in for by the time you finished pushing your over-sized grocery cart to the check-out lane?

None of these things were probably something you took note of at the time. However, they're all well-studied supermarket mind tricks to get you to buy more, says brand expert and consultant Martin Lindstrom in his books, *Buyology—Truth and Lies About Why We Buy*, and *Brandology—Tricks Companies Use to Manipulate Our Minds and Persuade Us To Buy*.

Here are 11 supermarket strategies I take in to consideration when shopping, and for you to be aware of:

• The cart is huge on purpose. The bigger the cart, the more you buy.

- Middle shelves home the worse of the bunch. They're within arms' reach for you to grab, and go.

- The good foods, generic and bulk items (cheaper) you need to work for. Typically, these are shelved high or low away from eye level or child appeal.

- Staples are hidden. Eggs and milk are intentionally placed in the back of the store to make you walk through the rest of the aisles to get there, potentially buying more along the way.

- End caps host nothing special. Marketers are simply paying more to double advertise in those spaces to catch your eye as you pass by. It's a method of "curb appeal" to be enticing from the perimeter.

- Options aren't always a good thing. Too many and your brain can't deal with processing all of the choices, let alone understand nutrition labels and marketing ploys.

- Small, crowded aisles entice you to buy fast and impulsively.

- Avoid the free samples, which are typically boxed, fake, or processed with ingredients you can't read.

- Like the music you hear? That's intentional. Feeling good when you shop means you buy more.

- Stocking up on fresh produce at the beginning of the store is great— if you stop there. However, this can psychologically lead you to buy something outside the healthy norm because you're more relaxed or feel better by getting the produce first.

- Did the smell of baked bread remind you of being a kid or something your mom used to make? Smells of baked goods and the deli are intentional, and sometimes not even real. Nostalgia tugs at your emotional response system—and adds to your shopping cart.

Get smarter than the system, simplify your foods, and purchase with a purpose.

31. NOURISH WITH A LIFESTYLE, NOT A DIET

D-I-E-T.

The four letter word that isn't a swear word but can carry more emotion than any $h*t, f**k, or a$$ tied together in one sentence. It's time to change that perspective. Here's a perspective that I've ingrained in to my head anytime I get an email with the latest fad diet, or see a post of a #latestdiethashtaghere on social media.

According to Merriam-Webster's dictionary, by definition, a diet is:

a : food and drink regularly provided or consumed a diet of fruits and vegetables a vegetarian diet

b : habitual nourishment links between diet and disease

c : the kind and amount of food prescribed for a person or animal for a special reason was put on a low-sodium diet

d : a regimen of eating and drinking sparingly so as to reduce one's weight going on a diet

As I mentioned in the opener of this chapter, diets are like dating. There are one-night-stands—the juice cleanse, the 1200 calories diet, cabbage soup diet—and then there are the ones you date to marry—#lifestylenotadiet. As a gal once divorced and now (happily) remarried, I've done the one-night-stands in the past throughout my eating disorder days. Now, and here in this section, I'm focused on the love-me-long-time diet.

So how do you shift the focus on creating a lifestyle when you're sleeping around with the diets?

Trial and error, baby. And understand that there are no fast fixes, pills, or quick weight-loss tips that will offer you a lifetime of health and well-being. Any form of a diet will have a short-term effect on your weight. When you change your meals, or eliminate one food, your body needs to adjust and you will see some of the benefits within a week or two, or sometimes even within a few days.

However, how long can you really eat just cabbage soup? Or, drink only juices? Worse, from my own experience, minimize your caloric intake? These are all short-term fixes, and in the end, most of the weight is gained back from water that was lost. After the cleanses and focusing on just the calories is a slippery slope that I've shared in Part 1 and 2 of this book to confirm that it's not a fix for caring for properly nourishing your body.

Your body isn't a thing, it's alive, and an action that is constantly changing and transforming. Make a lifetime commitment to your body, and look for the long-term solutions for a long healthy relationship with the one you need to love the most—YOU!

32. NOURISH WITH SELF-CARE

The saying goes, you never know what you've got till it's gone. And, damn, is that true when it comes to your health! As we've gone over in this book already, you can't prevent the world from happening, but you can do your very best to take the best care of YOU day in and day out to be healthy and nourished.

Here are 10 of my top self-care tips to work in to your day:

1. Sleep — we all have excuses why we can't get in our 8 hours. Just do your best, tick back your bedtime a few more minutes each night until you can achieve it, and there is no such thing as, "I'll make up for it on the weekend."

2. Wake up and stretch first thing — even 60 seconds of a side bend, back bend and twist stretch can change your morning.

3. Dry Brush — your skin is the largest living organ on your body, don't ignore it. Use a natural-bristle brush, on dry skin, and sweep it all up over your body, in the direction toward your heart. This gets the lymphatic system moving and speeds up draining and detoxification in the body. It also works great on reducing cellulite and water retention.

4. Drink plenty of water — Carry a water bottle around with you, drink filtered, pure, clean agua and let water be your first two drinks of every day (yes, even before coffee).

5. Make time everyday to do something just for you — Meditate in the morning, read a book, take a yoga class, cook your favorite meal, grab a coffee and people watch. Schedule YOU time in.

6. Stare out a window from time to time — who ever said daydreaming was a bad thing? I've had so many inspiring and creative moments occur while staring at the clouds or the planes that pass by my apartment overhead. It's good NOT to think every now and then to refresh your mental energy.

7. Immerse yourself in nature — We all have our unique happy place. Mine is the ocean, yours could be the mountains, or planting in your garden. Connect to Earth.

8. Hug someone — It can be a friend, your spouse, your son or daughter, your puppy, or even a (safe) stranger. Hugging can boost your feel-good endorphins.

9. _Moon, or silence, your phone throughout the day_ — The updates, messages, emails, and DINGS are incredibly distracting and can drain you of energy, removing your focus. Unless I know I have a scheduled call coming in, I'm in moon mode 24/7.

10. _Take a vacation_ — Book it. Pack your bags, pick a place, and just GO! Even better if it's a solo trip. We can work our entire lives, for... what? Get out, experience the world, learn a new language, or explore a new culture. You will return back home with a fresh perspective on life, and YOU, as a person.

33. NOURISH THROUGH EXPERIMENTATION

Growing up in Connecticut, I never would have guessed one day I'd be eating a cactus. Cacti are plants you stick in your window and water once every 2 or so weeks, right?

Never say never. Today, **_nopal_**, an edible cactus plant native to Mexico, is one of my favorite items to pick up from the farmers market once we land in Mexico City or the Riviera Maya in Quintana Roo. It has this slimy, gooey inside when you cut and cook it, but tastes absolutely delicious mixed in with tomatoes, zucchini, or topped with fresh avocado.

One of the things I appreciate about traveling is the opportunity to experiment with food. When I am traveling and cooking, I'm typically using far fewer ingredients than I would back at home. Or, I get a chance to test out foods that are new to me, but local to the lands, and have the opportunity to expand my palette and create a dish I would never be able to back at home. Had I only eaten what I knew from my usual meals, I never would have stumbled upon this delicious new food. Plus, it excites me to have something different, creating variety in my meals, rather than always eating the same. Same old can get boring fast.

Avoid the monotony of your dishes, and experiment with a fresh ingredient from time to time. While travel can certainly force you to do so, you don't necessarily have to travel to do this. Each week, pick up a new vegetable or fruit in the grocer you've never tried. Do some research, or Google, how to prep it. Add in to your meals trying out a few ways to prepare it (raw, cooked, boiled, baked, to name a few).

Eating what's in season can help you achieve variety and freshness as well. Although, these days, in the United States, thanks to preservation and imports, you can pretty much eat what you want when you want any time of the year. Learn what is in season prior to purchasing, or shop at a local farmer's market and inquire. Not only will you get what is freshest, but also typically buying what's in season can be cheaper as well.

34. NOURISH WITH QUALITY + QUANTITY

What you fear is what you manifest. When I was super focused on how many calories I was eating, I actually weighed more than I do now, I was far less happy in life and with myself, and the quality of the food I was eating was less than ideal. I feared gaining weight, being "fat" and being unhappy with myself. And, in fact, that's exactly how I felt. I was unhappy and heavier than my body was designed to be by trying to control an already perfectly functioning system.

How alive is the food you're eating, and what positive qualities are you bringing to your plate? By switching the focus on the quality of the food—going back to that idea of how "alive" the food is, and how fresh it tastes — rather than the focus on the calorie count, grams of fat, or portion of my plate, allowed me to enjoy, taste, and develop a relationship once again with food that nourished and fed me—literally, and emotionally.

Look at your plate like a canvas. How boring would your painting be if it was all beige and gray foods? Add some color! When you go to the grocery store, think of buying fresh produce like collecting paint swatches. When it comes time to prepare your meals, include a variety of hues and encourage your creativity come out when preparing your meal.

If you're working to change your eating habits for the better—focus your attention on what you're adding in, rather than what you're taking away. A slice of butter has 200 calories, but so does an entire plate filled with broccoli. The quality and quantity of the broccoli goes way farther than a tiny slab of dairy fat, not to mention the additional nutrients and vitamins you get from the plate of greens.

By focusing on the abundance of food you are adding in, you'll be less likely to focus on what you're taking away. Plus, who can complain about starving when you have an entire plate full of greens and veggies in front of you? Nourish yourself with quality, and let the quantity speak for itself.

35. NOURISH WITH WHY

Why do we eat when, or what, we eat? Is it because it's 12pm and that means lunchtime in our society? Or, are you really hungry? Are we having drinks and *tapas* after work because that's happy hour time? Or, perhaps we actually want that one drink because it tastes good?

Maybe this concept of questioning and pondering your why is new, but it can be a life-changing proposition to really empower your newer, healthier habits in the moments of question or doubt.

I didn't exactly know it at the time, but part of the reason I started my relationship with anorexia and bulimia was out of a need to numb the emotions that I wasn't able to acknowledge or process. I wanted control, and was solely focused on losing weight or the binge and purge cycle to get rid of the food I did consume. That was my WHY, for eating, or not eating.

It was the same reason when it came to drinking. I wanted to allow myself that freedom to let go, release, and be free from my own thoughts and feelings for those few hours while drinking and inebriation. It was the freedom to not think or do, but to just be—a form of unhealthy release I was seeking all of those years.

Today, when I eat, or select my meals, I am much more compassionate with myself as the WHY for eating is based on a long-term goal of health and well-being. If I'm feeling a bit sluggish, or my immune system is down, prior to making a meal, I strategize what foods I want to eat that will give me energy or boost my immunity.

Learning how foods affect you, as an individual, can help you better understand how to make foods work for you as an arsenal and toolkit, to give you the healthier benefits you're seeking. I've found it useful to keep a journal when starting out learning how different foods affect you, and your energy.

Observe how a food makes you feel before, during and after eating it. Does it leave you feeling anxious beforehand? Does it have a weird taste, or texture, in your mouth when chewing it? How does that food sit in your stomach after digesting? Do you want to run a marathon, or take a nap, after eating it?

Keep track of an arsenal of foods and see how they impact how you feel, and use that knowledge to your advantage. Those observations will greater serve you in the future when deciding what to eat and why you're eating it. When your why is for "health" and immunity, there will be no question that you'll choose the plate of greens for dinner over the oil-dipped french fries and greasy burger.

36. NOURISH WITH SELF-AWARENESS

Self-awareness is one of the first powerful steps towards creating change. If you're not aware of something, or that it's not working for you, how can you change it?

During my bulimia years, there were certain triggers, foods, or environments that I knew would set me off on a binge and purge cycle. Some examples: A Friday night alone, by myself in my apartment; A jar of open peanut butter; A box of cereal that would begin as one bowl, then another, then four more. All of these would lead to a binge/purge.

Observing and learning these triggers, with time, I was able to develop strategies to work around them. My goal was clear: stop throwing up. How did I make that happen? I planned ahead.

I made plans for Friday night to go out with a friend, paint my nails (you can't have wet nails and eat food or throw up), or commit to seeing a movie. I bought single serving sizes of peanut butter instead of an entire jar. I stopped eating cereal at night. I would only eat it as a morning meal or midday snack.

In this case, short-term fixes chosen based on self-awareness began to create lasting long-term habits. If you know certain times of the day or being in a particular environment is a trigger for you, develop tactics that you can implement that will make you feel good about you, the decisions you make, and encourage you towards achieving your goal of being healthier and more committed to you.

The other part of this concept is to nourish you. So, when creating those tactics, plan in something that is positive or healing for you. Not only will doing something for yourself send a positive message to your brain that, *"HEY! You're worth it and deserve this effort!"* but you'll further feel empowered by taking positive action towards healthier choices that you've committed yourself to.

37. NOURISH WITH SELF-TRUTH AND #OWNYOURWEIRD

Back in 2017, I had the opportunity to visit and document a private island off the coast of Fiji for a press trip. I was lucky to be able to bring a plus one, so Javier was able to join, film, and enjoy as well. This island was like a slice of Gilligan's eco-paradise, with private luxury *palapas*, a football field of solar panels, and even their own vegetation of fresh produce daily. I was in papaya and green salad heaven!

I was also the only vegan who chose not to drink in the entire group of 14. When you have a history of an eating disorder, group meal times can already be tricky. Being the only one not eating meat, dairy, wine and asking for special dishes in front of a group you know no one in? That can be a huge trigger for a former eating disordered individual.

Until I was reminded by Javi on one of the first days after a group lunch, *"Eh, so what if you are the only one not eating meat and you need to ask for exactly what you want. So what if it are three plates of papaya and fruits, and a double order of greens. Never settle right?"* Javi was right, and speaking the words right out of my own manifesto.

Here's where the phrase ***"Own Your Weird"*** came to life. It's the mantra I used at every meal gathering, and each time I needed to kindly ask the chef to make a special side order for the vegan in the crew who actually does eat, and eats a lot! She just has a few special dietary requests if he would be so kind to create.

By day three, the chef had my orders down pat, and I was getting some of the most delectable dishes out of the entire crew. Better yet, by the end of the trip, other writers and photographers from the press crew were openly sharing that my meal looked even better than theirs, and that they envied I was able to eat so healthy and well.

#lifestylenotadiet #ownyourweird

So, own what makes you unique, ask for what you want, and don't be afraid to make a special request from time to time. You deserve health, and you deserve what you want—weird, or not so weird.

~

For more information and recipes on the subjects of food and nutrition, refer to the resources page at https://saraquiriconi.com/book/resources/

↦

CHAPTER 12:
LIVING FREE + WITH PURPOSE

MAY 5, 2003, STRATFORD, CONNECTICUT

Flashback to 2003, and I'm reflecting back on an afternoon sitting at a Starbucks, drinking coffee, avoiding food, doing my college homework and making small talk. I was drumming up a conversation with a gentleman equally alone, yet graciously happy and fulfilled compared to my empty soul at the time.

"Today, someone said something that really made me think.

In reference to the weather, I commented on the misty rain that has been falling for the past few days to the man selling magazines, walking door to door. I said, 'Too bad you don't have better weather outside.' He replied, 'You know somethin', sista? I've walked in the pouring rain in the snow, the sleet, the hail, just to get my cocaine, heroine and otha drugs. To me, this is just liquid sunshine.'

"Liquid sunshine, I thought. Good perspective. The guy's been clean for three days. I understand his struggle. To others, three days is nothing; it sounds like three seconds.

For me, going three days without binging and purging, eating correctly, not feeling guilty, feeling healthy and normal: that would be a great feeling. Like liquid sunshine."

That feeling, that perspective, and that freedom of choice is what living free is based on. I know now all of the previous struggles I've learned, dealt with, and have overcome were all part of the greater plan and path to be present to share this message with you. I believe in you. I believe that you can overcome any obstacle in your life. It starts with awareness and action, but first—*CHOICE.*

The Big C can be a cancer, in many of its forms, as we've discussed throughout this book. However, the big C can be just as empowering if we flip the switch and call it a CHOICE. With responsibility and ownership of our lives and actions, we're no longer victims, but empowered warriors, on a path to CHOOSE our lives, our perspectives, and even our health.

38. CHANGE WHAT YOU CANNOT ACCEPT, OR ACCEPT WHAT YOU CANNOT CHANGE.

I'd be lying if I said you can change whatever you want in the world to make your life better. That's just not true, and that's not life. There are some things we can alter, physically, and other things we need to alter, mentally. It's about acceptance—of what we cannot change.

I couldn't change my cancer diagnosis after it was given. I couldn't get my job back after being laid-off. I couldn't just wake up one day and say *"Hey, Sara, let's stop throwing up today, please?"* I tried for years. It didn't work.

What I could change was my perspective on all of the above. The cancer diagnosis I saw as a challenge to overcome, not a death sentence. The job loss eventually pushed me in the direction towards yoga, and teaching, which helped me heal from the eating disorder. And not throwing up? Well, I can accept that my past has taught me a lot about valuing my health, my body, and the quality of food that I choose to put in to my body today. It has given me the power of mind to overcome anything, and the strength to ask for what I really want in life.

Start with one area in your life that you want to change. Write it down. Next, make two columns with the headings *"In Control"* and *"Free bird."*

What aspects surrounding this area do you have control over? Write those down under the *"In Control"* column. What is completely out of your hands? Write these reflections under the *"Free Bird"* category.

Make a separate note below of all this and write down your ideal outcome. What is your ultimate goal? What is the ideal scenario?

Now look at the *"In Control"* column and decide what steps you can take to move closer towards your goal located at the bottom. In other words, how does your problem trickle down to your goal/solution? Those are your actions to take. #noexcuses commit to making it happen.

Head to the *"Free Bird"* category and write down notes of how you can reframe or rephrase those topics in your mind to make peace with them. If you're a control freak like me, this is where the hard work comes into play. This can require more effort because it's conscious or unconscious thoughts or beliefs that you need to rewire in your brain.

Keep this list handy, for the moments you're in turmoil or in the same situation to refer back to your WHY and keep pushing towards that goal at the bottom of your list.

Not only does this strategy empower you to take action, but it also frees you from feeling like a victim or being stuck in a circumstance you aren't particularly fond of.

39. TAKE ACTION FROM HEART, NOT FROM EXPECTATION TO OUTCOME.

This happens many mornings in my household. I'm up early, rise and shine, putting away the dishes from the night before and making the coffee for us. My husband stumbles downstairs and mutters a 'Good morning, love' barely awake. I stand there, infuriated, by his lack of effort to see all that I've done in the morning for us, and not even the slightest mention of a thank you!

Poor guy, I know. He needs a bit more time in the morning than me to wake up. And over time, I've learned, that if I do something, from the heart, and because I want to do it, not because I was expecting something from it then I need to accept this morning routine (and not begrudge Javi). This example is a small piece of greater inner turmoil we drum up in our minds about action and expectation. However, it's a small glimpse of perhaps a relatable example of how we interact with others and our minds on a daily basis.

The same outlook can apply to social media, your job, favors for friends, and raising your children. What are you offering, sharing, or doing for someone else (followers, your boss, a friend, your kids) and what are you seeking? Knowing your why, and being clear that you're doing something because it serves YOU before anyone can free you from the disappointment and expectation that you may have felt if you did something just for the sake of someone else's pleasure.

Share a post on social media—not for the likes or follows, but—because it's an expression of you, your message and your emotion.

Do something in your job, or express an idea to a boss—not just for the recognition and raise, but—because of your pride, intelligence, and expertise.

Offer to help a friend—not to have a you owe me, on your friend for the future, but—because it feels good doing something for someone else from a place of love.

When you're acting from the heart, and from what leaves you feeling good, you won't be as attached to the expectation, freeing you from that entrapment of anger, hurt, and disappointment.

40. IF YOU DON'T WANT TO BE TREATED LIKE A NUMBER, STOP OPERATING LIKE ONE.

Repeat after me, or read these words out loud:

I am not a paycheck.

I am not a weight.

I am not a follower count.

I am not a zip code.

I am not a car model.

These numbers may seem incredibly important right now, in your life, but ten years from now, or during your last days on this Earth, they will certainly be insignificant and meaningless. Life will treat you how you see yourself. And, if you see yourself defined by these numbers, you will be treated that same exact way in return.

Instead of basing your life on numbers, emphasize the feelings that arise from each of them. How does the job your receiving that paycheck from make you feel? How does your body allow you to feel and move and experience life? How does the ability to reach a mass of millions, or maybe 70, followers empower you to share something worthwhile and impactful in this world? Do you feel connected, and at ease, in the current home you reside in? And, does your car leave you with the freedom to move and get to be places you need to without leaving you in a pile of debt?

Values, by definition, can be a number. But on a deeper level, develop your values for life. It may sound heavy to think about, but imagine you were given a week to live. In reality, none of us really knows when our last day is, so perhaps this question is more a reality-check of our mortality than it is a heavy topic.

If you were given a week to live, what you pack into that week doing? Who would you see? What activities would you do? What foods would you eat? What actions would you take?

There are exhaustive lists of values on the Internet,,ones you can find by doing a simple search. Google "List of Values" and pick on that has 50-200 to base your search on. From that list, select and write down any that resonate with you. Refine, edit, and whittle that list down, eventually, to five values that truly define and resonate with you who you are—authentically, happily, and truthfully.

This list of five core values can help you shape, take action on, and develop your day-to-day life. In the end, literally and figuratively, you'll be happier, fulfilled, and feeling complete from a life well lived.

41. COLLECT EXPERIENCES OVER THINGS.

Shopping for material things is an emotional experience. One that has us looped in the moment of instant gratification and the idea that if we buy just this one thing, this item, then our lives will transform, where we'll all of sudden be happy, healthy, perfect and complete from the benefits and gratification from this one item.

Even though this may sound a bit dramatic, that is actually the psychology behind advertising and marketing to consumers. The *"I need to buy this now and then I will be happy and healthy!"* mentality is the goal of each TV commercial, online ad, email newsletter sale, and social media promo. What happens when that moment after purchase passes?

The same hole of feeling empty or lacking is still left with you, and you're quickly searching for the next quick fix to feel that high again.

Before you go all monk on me and sell off all of your possessions and donating the rest to Goodwill, get excited about becoming a minimalist and a realist at the same time. I, for one, would be lost without some of my cameras, laptop, hard drives and headphones. I'm a tech junkie who likes nice things that allow me to create and share. I love my bed, my pillows, fluffy sheets and towels, and soft cotton PJs to sleep in. I buy quality fruits, vegetables, and sprouted grains to eat well and maintain my health.

None of these are in excess, they're things I need to live the life I want. What I don't need? The extra clothes, the latest iPhone, the best silverware and dish sets, or a high-end dining room table. I don't even own a dining room table, because we prefer to eat seated cross-legged on a carpet and cushions with a low table (it's better for your hips and posture, anyway).

My personal motto: I spend where I need to and save for the adventures. I know that traveling, seeing new places, taking incredible photos and videos from those trips, are all things that I will remember and create memories for a lifetime. I spend on education, trainings, books, and online tutorials that keep my brain fresh, creative, active, and always learning. I spend on my health, but within limits (I refuse to spend $10 on a juice, but I have no problem buying four cantaloupes for the same amount to eat throughout the week).

Save where you can, and spend on what fuels you for a lifetime. Develop a list of those *life fuels*, and put your efforts and savings towards those experiences that will fulfill you long past an "add to cart and buy" material purchase.

42. DON'T SURVIVE. THRIVE.

Cancer Survivor: this title happens from the moment you are diagnosed with cancer, through your treatment and stays with you for life thereafter. I, personally, didn't think of myself as a survivor until after the treatment was finished and I was told I was officially cancer free. Defining this phrase, then, seems to be a personal preference.

Either way, I was never truly a fan of the word "survivor" to encapsulate how I wanted to live after cancer. By definition, survivor is *"to remain alive or in existence: to live on"* (Merriam-Webster's Dictionary). While there's nothing wrong with the word survivor, I feel like it leaves us a bit short of our potential to take all the lessons we can from such life-changing events.

Change a few letters, switch up the order, and I use the term *"cancer thriver"* instead. Simply surviving, to me, seemed a bit more of the victim mentality, as if you were lucky or only by chance still alive. When we can thrive, after any momentous event, such as cancer, a loss, a divorce, overcoming addiction, or any "aha" moment, there are so many more lessons we can pull from that tragedy life has given us—with reason.

Life presents us with situations, hardships, challenges, and experiences from which we can learn something. As I've mentioned before, we're not victims of life, we're warriors learning, growing and rising through it. How does the difficult circumstance in front of you offer a chance to learn something or to grow?

All of the "super powers" I feel I have today to live a life I dream, to leap without being stuck in fear, and to act from intuition is in many thanks to all that you've read about in Parts 1 and 2 of this book. But in reality, there's nothing super about my powers—it's about thriving.

Shift from being a victim, a survivor just getting by through luck, and find ways you can learn and grow in any circumstance that will encourage you to thrive.

43. NEVER TRY. NEVER KNOW.

Think of a time or an opportunity that has been placed in front of you. It's new, it's a challenge and, maybe, it's something you haven't done before or know exactly how to succeed at. Now think how long it took you to answer, "Yes" or "No" to accepting this opportunity. Before you can even answer, your mind has probably already unconsciously decided for you whether you will succeed or not succeed. What is the power in knowing that? Henry Ford said it best:

"Whether you think you can, or you think you can't—you're right."

What if's? and regrets can be a form of mental tumor if you let them run off on a tangent. The remorse one feels and the negative side effects on a person for not taking action to do something can be far greater than if one had tried and failed miserably. At least you would know the outcome, or have learned something along the way.

When I'm making decisions in such moments, I play out the game of **"worst case scenario."** If you're contemplating trying something new, write out three different possible outcomes. One will be exactly what you hope for. Another, the absolute worst, most terrible, shit-hits-the-fan, kind of scenario. The other, will fall somewhere in between the previous two. If any one of these outcomes occur simply by you trying, what is the worst that could happen, really?

You want a raise. You ask your boss, and the worst case, he fires you. OK, you can find another job. Best case, he says yes. The in-between outcome is he says no, or requests you to come up with a list of reasons why you have earned a raise.

You want to overcome your desire to binge eat tonight, trying to drown your sense of emptiness. Worst case, it doesn't happen and you overeat once again. Try again tomorrow. Best case, you call a friend, do your nails, have a small snack in between, and feel full that evening in a different, heart-felt way.

Two very different scenarios, but understanding the point that when you can work out the potential outcomes, often times you'll see that had you never tried in the first place, you'd never know the potential to learn from the outcome. A life without regrets is one of the most freeing feelings you can experience.

44. TIME IS ENERGY, ENERGY IS CURRENCY—AND TIME IS THE MOST VALUABLE THING YOU HAVE.

Money, you can make more of. Time, you can never get that back. Not even Jeff Bezos (founder of Amazon, and at this time, the wealthiest person alive) can buy more time on this Earth. The higher powers of our Universe don't accept money deals, and they certainly don't accept payoffs. And, when you pass away, any of the money you've acquired, you can't take with you.

In that case, the only thing you can really place a value on is your time.

What are you giving your time to in this one life? Who are you giving your energy to? What is worth your personal value and currency? And, in that matter, what value are you placing on yourself? Is it high enough? Do you need to up your currency value?

Imagine the time and energy of your day, collectively. Put that "value" into the form of a trading stock on the market. What is the value of your stock? This number can't come from anyone else but you—and make it high! You're a blue chip stock, warriors; not some penny trade.

Now, as you're "trading" your stock with other interactions throughout your day, be sure your trade is giving you the optimal return on investment, or ROI. Get back what you give, and if not, trade elsewhere.

A consistently stressful job, draining conversations, negative thought patterns—these all can be bad trades and interactions. How can we trade up, and invest our stocks higher? Shift and find other transactions to take part of that leave you feeling more fulfilled, increasing your value, and, in return, give you the greatest form of reward you can receive: health, happiness, passion and purpose.

45. PLAY MORE. THINK LESS.

Why, as kids, do we push to grow up so fast? Then, as adults, we seek freedom to be a kid again. Doubt me? Two "V" words to consider: Video games and Vegas.

I'm starting a new trend: 4 is the new 30, and 6 is the new 40. Read that again if you need to to understand it. *4 is the new 30, and 6 is the new 40.* If I can suggest any magic potion to be the fountain of youth, I'd offer that it is **PLAY.** When we allow ourselves to plan, and get out of our rationalizing, thinking mind, that's where we delve into creativity and passion. That point where we get lost in just being, and having fun, is where we can not only feel youthful and playful, but we can rewire our brains to develop new connections and to relieve stress.

So, let's play! What were some of the things you used to love doing as a kid that you no longer do as an adult? Where is there some time in your calendar that you can implement FREE and PLAY time to go outdoors, learn a new skill, play with a puppy, or even spend some time around the best teachers for this segment: KIDS.

Age is simply a number. What matters is how we're spending that time, those years, and those moments. Stress and over-thinking will age us and wear us down. Play can clear some of that weight, and free our spirits, and keep us feeling young, no matter the number of candles on that birthday cake you have to blow out each year.

46. REPLACE THE WORDS "SHOULD" AND "HAVE-TO" WITH "OPPORTUNITY" AND "CHOICE."

Starting a sentence with "should" is like starting a conversation with "don't"—it's off-putting, negative, and we immediately feel adverse or wrong in some way for our previous actions.

It's a terrible feeling, but it's also one we allow ourselves to take on. "Should" is one of my least favorite words in the English language. In fact, I strive my hardest to not use the word in any of my conversations or sentences, because I know how that word makes me feel. The word should and have-to is like putting ourselves back in that 8-year old mindset where we did something wrong and now we're being corrected for it or told what to do. If we accept that fate, then we're going with the status quo, doing what society has told us, settling for average and running on the hamster wheel of what is accepted, or expected.

Boring. And you will feel bored with that at some point, after a while of doing the "shoulds"—or worse, resentful. Throughout our lives, we're told shoulds and have-to's all the time from external sources, in an effort to change, or guide, our behavior:

"You should get a full time job in finance."

"You should become a doctor."

"You have to have a kid."

"You have to clean your plate."

All of these sentences are fairly harmless in the moment; however, over time they can ingrain another form of thinking that creates negative habits that we're doing unconsciously. The next time you feel like you should or have to do something, pause for a moment and hear your own words in your head. Where are they really coming from? Is it from a parent who used to say that to you when you were a kid? Is it a teacher that taught you something years ago in grade school?

Even further, be OK with giving yourself the space to close your eyes for a few moments and visualize, where is this voice actually coming from? Who is the author of this voice? What does the voice sound like? What age am I? Where are you in that observant situation?

Who is really the person doing the talking and guiding? If it isn't you, cut that voice out, and listen to the only source and guide that will know what you should or have to do, and that's your intuition.

As a visual strategy, wear a bracelet or a band reminding yourself to filter out the limiting words and beliefs. Write on a rubber-band the word "CHOICE" to wear on your wrist. As you see that word throughout the day, it's a reminder anytime the word *should* or *have-to* pops up in conversation or in your mind.

Take it a step further and see if you can remove the words should and have to from your own vocabulary and conversations with others. See how it feels to empower the other person to make their own decision. You may find yourself to be a better listener, guide and friend because of it.

Remember, every action is a choice. The sooner you realize and accept that responsiblity, you'll be one step closer towards living FREE.

47. JUST START, AND KEEP MOVING FORWARD.

I'm a closet hockey fan, so this one comes from the ice legend and Hall of Famer, Wayne Gretzky:

"You miss 100% of the shots you don't take."

Fear can be the greatest blocker for our ability to change. Even if we know the change would be for the better, there are an insurmountable number of fears that could prevent us from ever even trying to think in a different way, let alone try it. Here's a quick list of steps to get you thinking, and taking action, to shift from "I Can't" to "I Am Trying":

1. *Begin with your WHY, or your desire.* Write down what exactly you want to achieve from this change. (I've always wanted to try cooking classes.)

2. *Take a safe, small step forward.* If you know you have nothing to lose, it doesn't hurt to try in any capacity. Choose an action that can take you one bit closer towards your goal that you know you will lose nothing by exploring. (Google search online courses and local courses you can take in your area—most cities offer community programs. Call a few to find out dates and pricing.)

3. *Child's pose it. Reflect. Observe.* How do you feel after taking that step forward? Did you come any closer towards where you want to be? Do you still want to pursue your goal? (Yes! They have a weekend class for smoothie making I will take on my free day.)

4. *Practice makes practice.* Repeat the above steps, until your will to try overcomes your will to "I can't because..." There's no perfect course, just your own journey.

So, get in front of that goal, grab your stick, and slap the puck. Whether you make a goal, ding off a post, or miss the shot entirely. That doesn't matter. Just starting, trying, and getting over that initial fear can be the biggest leap you need to eventually succeed.

48. NEVER SETTLE.

When was the last time you said "OK" to something just to make life easier? What stood in your way of asking for something different? Was it a fear? The effort? A confrontation? Potential conflict?

Life is full of those pivotal moments where we can either sink back and simply go with the flow, or we can swim upstream and make the effort to go in the direction our hearts truly sing for.

On the trip to Playa del Carmen to write the first two parts of this book, I moved rooms four times in the first hotel, until finally asking for a refund and changing hotels—all in the same afternoon. The first room had a terrible leak in the ceiling with water dripping in, and the next two did as well. The last room was facing the ocean, and with the borderline tropical storm that was passing through, I knew that my light-sleeper self wouldn't be able to get a wink of shut-eye with the shutters and door slamming.

I went to the front desk, and kindly explained my situation and frustration and need for peace on this trip. There's always a kind way, and a not so nice way, to ask for what you want—the former will get you further. I requested a refund, and explained that I would be moving to another hotel that evening. With fantastic customer service, they understood, and processed my refund, wishing me to revisit on an upcoming opportunity to experience how wonderful we both knew this resort is under regular weather conditions. We both left happy, feeling good about the interaction.

And me? I had a blissful night sleep in the other hotel. Peace and a sound structure at the five-star accommodation gave me comfort. I knew I needed quiet, I knew I needed a safe environment, and I knew I wanted my rest to be my best for writing this book. Was it an effort to spend all afternoon changing rooms and explaining my story? Yes. Was it a pain to pack and unpack my bags four times in the matter of 5 hours? Heck yeah. And, was it a hassle to pay multiple cabs, charging double the accommodation fees to my credit card while the refund was processing? CitiBank concurs, absolutely.

In the end, it was all worth it. I knew that my extra effort to ask kindly and get what I needed was going to be worth any challenge to overcome in the long run.

We often settle in many areas in our lives to avoid the effort or the conflict. Jobs keep us steady, relationships prevent us from being alone, and pills numb the physical pain. But here's where we need to be honest with ourselves. Are we really happy in that space and receiving what we need? Or, are we just settling?

Only you can make that honest call, warriors. However, if it's settling, I encourage you to:

...Ask for that raise!

...To tell your partner what you really need in your relationship together.

...Get to the root of your physical pain, **UNFCK Your Body*** and reduce your pain medications, or get rid of them all together!

Because life—it's too short to just settle. Get what you want, and be willing to put in the muscle to do the work to make it happen. No one else will do it for you, but YOU.

49. QUALITY OVER QUANTITY.

In terms of living well, bigger doesn't mean better, and more doesn't equate to happiness. Ask any millionaire or billionaire, money doesn't make you happy—how you live with it will. The late Notorious B.I.G.

* *UNFCK Your Body is a movement methodology designed to heal and restore one's body back to it's balanced range of motion. Created by Sara Quiriconi, Live Free Warrior, this series can be practiced and downloaded ondemand here: https://vimeo.com/ondemand/unfckyourbody or from the resource page at https:// saraquiriconi.com/book/resources/*

said it best: *"Mo Money, Mo Problems."*

I've always joked, a bigger home only means more bathrooms to clean. True, if someone is wealthy enough to own a mansion, that person probably has the funds to hire housekeeping help. Sarcasm and logistics to the side, you get the point.

Having more of something won't make you happy, nor will it make you healthy. In fact, the opposite can be true, where too much of anything is never a good thing. I can promise you that from my alcoholic days.

My immediate family and I live on opposite sides of the East Coast. We don't get a chance to see each other often; however, when we do, we are sure to cherish the time to the fullest. The quality of the time we spend is far greater than the quantity.

The same goes for the food you eat. Eating more greens and veggies won't make you healthier, if they're covered in cream dressing or doused with pesticide spray. The quality of food you put in to your body is a key factor to focus on, over the quantity that you're taking in. That's a solid point I like to emphasize when talking about calories as well.

I spent so many years focusing on the quantity of calories I was consuming. What I didn't stop to focus on was the quality of the calories. I should have been focused on: were the foods I was eating free from GMO's, toxic additives, fake dyes, unnatural sweeteners, and other gene-altering chemicals.

Next time you're thinking of wanting MORE, consider focusing on the QUALITY of what you already have in front of you instead. Reflect on what you're in need of, then what's in front of you, and how you can be resourceful to make more of what you have instead of Costco-sizing your life in every aspect.

50. IF YOU WANT TO CHANGE THE WORLD, YOU FIRST NEED TO START WITH CHANGING YOURSELF.

The victim mentality is something I have zero patience for. The other one is blame. Both get you nowhere and leave you feeling miserable and, eventually, alone and angry.

The longer you point the finger at what others are doing wrong and what they need to change, the farther you'll be from connecting to the person who can actually make a change in anything—YOU.

Next time you start to seek reason or rationale from an external source or force, first see where there is an opportunity for you to take personal responsibility. What can YOU do for you right in this moment? What previous actions have you feeling the way you do right now? And, to what small degree or reason, did you assist in getting yourself to where you are in this moment?

In any relationship or scenario, it's a two way street. To some capacity, there is a small part you can take action on. But, being able to take action on anything first requires awareness, then responsibility, and then freedom. Freedom comes from knowing you cannot change anyone else, nor their actions, but the ones you choose only for yourself. So, start there. Then, lead by example.

51. THE BEST BOOK IN THE WORLD IS A PASSPORT FULL OF STAMPS.

I was recently asked in an interview, if I could recommend what to do to any 25-year old who felt stuck, bored in life, or in need of a transition, what would it be? My answer was immediate, and one word: *Travel.*

Pack your bags, pick a destination, and just go! There are bonus points if you do this trip solo, and even better if it's to a place you've never been or is completely different than your daily way of living. What you will experience during that time, the people you will meet, interact with, the culture you can explore, to see how other people live—this will all change you. It's a change that you cannot learn in a book, nor is it something you come close to liking, commenting, or watching on social media.

The kind of value, life experiences, and understanding of the world around you is truly one of a kind, and the more you get out there and connect with the world around you, the more you'll begin to realize just how alike and similar we are—as humans—we all are. We want happiness, to be healthy, and to be loved. We all have our bad days, deal with family issues, have a negative boss, or can find something about our body we don't like. Being human isn't unique.

When you return from a transformational travel adventure, (something I experience on every trip I take) you'll never return home the same. With a fresh mindset, new skills, and a stirred perspective, an answer, idea, or direction will come to you when you upon your return. Being stuck is impossible when you chose to move.

52. YOU HAVE THE POWER TO CHOOSE ANY LIFE YOU DESIRE TO LIVE.

"Learn the rules like a pro, so you can break them like an artist." — *Pablo Picasso*

The tools and tips I outline in this book are just that: a starting point to learn some "rules," to test out what works best for you, leave behind what doesn't, and then make your own life tools or manifesto—now, as a *pro* of your own life, your own living free, and your own destiny.

Your life is a blank book and you are the author writing the story. There's no one else who will type the words, create the tale, develop the character, or resolve the conflict but you. Along your path, you will uncover many twists, you will discover many characters, and you will find yourself in many conflicts that test your will. However, strength and determination will help you to keep fighting to move forward. There may not be a happily ever after. All we know, dear warriors, is that the chapters of our lives are like artwork: never finished, only abandoned. And the words, allow them to flow: from the heart, from passion, from courage, from love, and from living freely each and every day like it's your last.

The Big C, the big CHOICE, is always yours to take on. And in terms of the Big C, meaning Cancer, while it may have the power to destroy the body, it can never destroy your soul. That is the power only you have, deep from within, to live life the way you wish to its best, healthiest and fullest.

To my live free warriors, may you be left with the inspiration now to live each and every one of your days writing the pages of your own book from this place of courage and power to *Live Cancer Free.*

ACKNOWLEDGEMENTS

The title of this book came to me in an instant, walking back from the beach one afternoon in Miami, from a mental voice that said, *"Living {Cancer} Free."*

The idea to write this book took 5 or so years, after meeting many new faces, opening up more about my past, healing bad habits and personal issues, and after hearing the conversations that repetitively ended, *"You should write a book. You can inspire millions."*

The lessons, reflections and content of this book, however, took 35 years—my entire life. There were many moments where the dark looked more promising than the light, where a cave and hiding was my way to cope and deal, and fear and anxiety had the ability to take over my mind.

Like a pyramid, a warrior's strength doesn't come from the peak of the structure, but from the power of its foundation. I want to thank the following individuals who have been my foundation, and supported, inspired and helped me make this book, my health and my life a reality:

First and foremost, thank you to my husband, my twin soul, Javier. Every day you challenge me, support me, bring me joy and give me the space to be ME. There is no crazier soul, or minion, I would want to spend this journey of life with other than you. #risinginlove

Thank you to my parents, for dealing with my shit for so many years, and having the heart, patience and strength to love, support and believe in me endlessly. Be proud—your girl is happy, strong and only getting better each day. You taught me we have the power to change something if we don't like it in our lives, and this book is exactly that. I love you.

Thank you to my brother, who is a quiet force in the family, yet stable, grounded, a light and a hidden strength. From the day you were born, I couldn't have been happier to have a brother to share memories and love with. I'm sorry for making you play dress up for all those years.

To my Great Aunt Helen, thank you for always being an example and inspiration to a life well lived, and of one lived freely.

To my editor, thank you, Beka Shayne Denter, for seeing the potential in me, this book and my message before I even had the vision. You are a strong, inspiring woman and the world needs more people like you in it.

To Leigh Weingus, thank you for your keen eye and insightful mind to review this book prior to launch—and for dealing with my typos.

Thank you to Marco, for believing in me when I didn't believe in myself. For being the inspiration at the time I needed it the most, to do the work on myself to become a better version of the life I wanted to live. And, for being the best Pup-Dad Pepina could have ever wanted.

AKNOWLEDGEMENTS

To Patrick, for being there in one of the most physically challenging times in my life through cancer. For having the courage to stand by someone going through such turmoil and not walk away. That takes heart.

To Len (whose name has been changed), you know who you are. Thank you for being a light in the darkness of my youth, and allowing me the space to just be me and free in a time I had no clue who I was.

Thank you to my Grandfathers, who are watching down on me from whatever universe or heaven you, the reader, believe in. I know I am on this path, guided by your lights and forces to lead a powerful movement to inspire millions that there is a freer, happier, healthier way.

Finally, thank you to you the reader, the listener, the fellow warrior, who is taking the time to do the work, who is seeking knowledge to become a better human, for yourself—and this world—and for being a drop of water in the ocean of positive change for living {cancer} free.

RESOURCES

Referenced throughout this book are a variety of resources available to you to support and guide you on your Live Free journey.

All, and more, of these resources can be found on the web-page:

https://saraquiriconi.com/book/resources/

On this book resource page, you will find:

FITNESS LINKS

- The complete UNFCK Your Body™ Video Series

- Yoga and Fitness Videos

BREATHWORK AUDIO EXERCISES (INCLUDING THOSE MENTIONED IN THIS BOOK)

- Inhale/Hold/Exhale Hold (p. 193)

- Clearing Space (p. 194)

- Relaxation Exercise (p. 195)

MEDITATION AUDIO EXERCISES (INCLUDING THOSE MENTIONED IN THIS BOOK)

- Body Scan (p. 198)

- Mirror On The Wall (p. 199)

- Hand Mantras (p. 200)

MUSIC REFERENCES

- Connecting to Silence (p. 211)

- Live Free Warrior Spotify Playlists (p. 205)

FOOD AND NUTRITION

- Superfoods (What are they? Why we need them? Where to try?)

- Healthy Food Recipes

- Live Free Warrior's Must-Have foods, part of the #lifestylenotadiet

ADDITIONAL RECOMMENDED RESOURCES

- Book References

- Movies of Inspiration and Research

- Holly Butcher's Full, Original Media Post

- Public Speaking Events or Retreats to Attend

- Connect Directly with Live Free Warrior, Sara Quiriconi